GET ALL THE ANSWERS
BEFORE YOU TRY MELATONIN

MELATONIN: The Anti-Aging Hormone details complete, scientific explanations on how this natural hormone works to keep the human body healthier longer.

Find out:

- What is melatonin?
- Why do researchers call melatonin the master hormone?
- Who should take melatonin supplements?
- Is melatonin safe?
- How does melatonin help the body in so many ways?

. . . and much more.

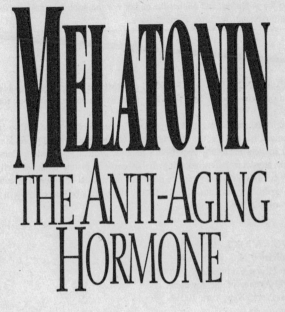

MELATONIN
THE ANTI-AGING HORMONE

SUZANNE LeVERT

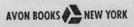

AVON BOOKS ◆ NEW YORK

MELATONIN: THE ANTI-AGING HORMONE is an original publication of Avon Books. This work has never before appeared in book form.

The ideas, procedures, and suggestions in this book are intended to supplement, not replace, the medical advice of a trained medical professional. All matters regarding your health require medical supervision. Consult your physician before adopting the suggestions in this book, as well as any condition that may require diagnosis or medical attention. The author and publisher disclaim any liability arising directly or indirectly from the use of this book.

AVON BOOKS
A division of
The Hearst Corporation
1350 Avenue of the Americas
New York, New York 10019

Copyright © 1995 by Suzanne LeVert
Published by arrangement with the author
Library of Congress Catalog Card Number: 95-94265
ISBN: 0-380-78304-5

First Avon Books Printing: October 1995

AVON TRADEMARK REG. U.S. PAT. OFF. AND IN OTHER COUNTRIES, MARCA REGISTRADA, HECHO EN U.S.A.

Printed in the U.S.A.

RA 10 9 8 7 6

Contents

Foreword

The late twentieth century represents a very exciting era in the history of medicine. At the same time that modern western medical technology has advanced to the point where it is able to explore the most minute and elusive cellular behavior, we as a society are beginning to reach a new understanding of the true meaning of health. Finally, physicians, their patients, and the general public equate health with feeling good—with energy, vitality, and the ability to appreciate life to its fullest—rather than merely the absence of disease.

In other cultures, particularly those of eastern religious traditions, the state known as health has long been connected to the idea of balance—balance within our bodies and between ourselves and the rest of the natural world. As the twenty-first century approaches, more and more of the world's citizens are beginning to appreciate once again the interdependence that exists among all living things, from microscopic organisms to human beings. Balance between our needs and the needs of the larger environment must be maintained in order for life as we know it to continue.

On an internal, cellular level, the same kind of interdependence appears to exist. Biochemists, physicians, and patients alike are starting to understand the linkage between each component of our anatomy and each function of our physiology—how the disruption of just one chemical or molecular task can undermine the health of our entire body.

In *Melatonin: The Anti-Aging Hormone*, author Suzanne LeVert takes you on a journey through the human body in order to show how one chemical, a hormone called melatonin, influences your health and vitality. As you'll see, melatonin appears to have remarkable effects on a wide variety of physiological activities, including the body's ability to rejuvenate itself with sleep, protect its cells from free radical damage, and bolster its ability to destroy bacteria, viruses, and even cancer cells.

Of all of melatonin's qualities, however, it is its influence on the body's internal clock that appears to have the most profound and widespread effects on our well-being. Recent research shows that melatonin may be the body's metronome—its rhythm-setter and rhythm-keeper—in charge of organizing and moderating all of its chemical, physical, emotional, and intellectual activities. On a daily basis, melatonin helps us to know when to wake and when to sleep, and helps other chemicals digest the food we eat, process the images we see, and work the muscles we move about. Over a lifetime, this powerful chemical may be responsible for triggering puberty, setting sexual and reproductive cycles in motion, stimulating brain activity, taking us through the aging process, and finally, leading us to death.

The study of body rhythms and their relationships to health and disease, chronobiology, is one of the fastest-growing and most fascinating fields of research in all of science. It shows us that the connection between time, nature, and the human body remains intact and is, in fact, integral to the way we function. Despite the fact that so much of our daily lives are now controlled by technology—by powers outside of nature and devoid of natural rhythm—it seems clear that our health is profoundly influenced by such "primitive" forces as sunshine and darkness, heat and cold, dampness and aridity.

Every day, we learn more about these natural rhythms—set in motion by the movement of the sun and the changing of the seasons—and the influence they have over all aspects of human physiology and behavior. As you'll soon discover, the practice of medicine has already begun to consider the implications outlined by chronobiology. It is now clear, for instance, that the action of certain drugs appears to improve depending on the time of day or year they are administered. As more becomes known about body rhythms, as well as melatonin's role in this fascinating aspect of human physiology, we will begin to include the impact of natural rhythms and cycles in discussions of health and disease.

In the meantime, as a doctor trained in both western and eastern philosophies of medicine, it is gratifying for me to see Americans looking for more natural ways to prevent disease, treat illnesses, and promote health—methods that attempt to attain and maintain balance, both internally and between man and the rest of nature. In this book, you'll find no "miracle cures" for aging or disease, nor will you be given any hard and fast rules or prescriptions. Instead, you'll learn about your body and the conditions under which it will best be able to stay healthy and stay well. Eating a nutritious diet, exercising on a regular basis, and avoiding toxic substances in the environment are a few of the proven ways to protect against disease and delay the onset of aging. Another way is to keep your body supplied with this essential substance, which you'll learn more about by reading *Melatonin: The Anti-Aging Hormone.*

—Glenn S. Rothfeld, M.D., M.Ac.
Clinical Instructor, Spectrum Medical Arts
Department of Family Medicine,
Tufts University School of Medicine

• 1 •

Melatonin:
The Master Hormone

What is melatonin?

Melatonin is a body chemical called a hormone that appears to have important and positive effects upon almost every system of the human body. Virtually every living organism, from one-celled amoeba to man, produces melatonin. However, our natural supply of the hormone is limited. After reaching a peak just before adolescence, melatonin levels drop with each passing year.

Fortunately, melatonin now is available in pill form to supplement and bolster natural production. Melatonin supplements appear to be relatively free from even minor side effects, are inexpensive, and are available without a prescription at health-food stores or through mail-order distributors across the country.

Why is melatonin important?

Long recognized as a potent sleep-promoting agent, researchers now link melatonin to a host of other potential health-enhancing properties. In addition to helping to reduce the effects of jet lag and curing all but the most intransigent cases of insomnia, melatonin is found to be a strong antioxidant, a stimulator of the immune system, and a natural pain-killer. Its use as an anti-cancer agent, a birth-control method, and a youth-enhancing formula are currently the subject of intense investigation in laboratories around the world.

Furthermore, melatonin appears to be an essential piece in a puzzle that has fascinated mankind since the dawn of time: Is there an internal mechanism that governs the life cycle of men and women? How is it that we develop and mature in such orderly and predictable patterns? What triggers the body to begin its decline into illness and old age? Are there ways to extend health and vitality past the current life-expectancy parameters? Through research on melatonin and other related physiological substances and mechanisms, we come closer every day to finding the answers to these and other intriguing questions.

Where does melatonin come from?

The main source of melatonin is the pineal gland, a tiny pine-cone shaped endocrine (hormone-secreting) organ located at the back of the brain just above the brain stem. Until recently, most scientists thought that the pineal gland was a vestigial organ—an organ that no longer plays a significant part in human physiology. Now that the essential functions of its major product, melatonin, have been identified, more attention is being paid to the pineal gland and its role in keeping the body and brain healthy and sound.

Is melatonin produced anywhere else in the body?

In addition to the pineal gland, melatonin has been found in a variety of other tissues. It is believed that the retina, the light-sensitive membrane that lines the eye, also produces melatonin. Another organ that appears to secrete melatonin is the large intestine, apparently in response to the amount and type of food that we eat.

How does what we eat affect how much melatonin we produce?

Melatonin, whose chemical name is N-acetyl-5-methoxyserotonin, is a derivative of a substance called tryptophan. Tryptophan is an amino acid, one of twenty-two organic compounds that are the basic building blocks of human life. Amino acids act as regulators of vital body activities—such as those that trigger the production of hormones like melatonin—as well as constitute the primary ingredients of muscles, bones, and other tissues.

The human body does not make tryptophan. Instead, tryptophan is one of eight "essential amino acids" that must be obtained from the diet. It is found in foods high in protein, especially legumes, grains, and seeds. A diet rich in those foods seems to influence the production of melatonin and other body chemicals.

How does tryptophan become melatonin?

Once digested, tryptophan is first synthesized into a substance called serotonin. Through a complex molecular process, serotonin is later converted into melatonin by the pineal gland when certain environmental and chemical signals reach that part of the brain.

Serotonin itself is a powerful neurotransmitter, a chemical that sends messages to and from nerve cells within the brain and throughout the body. As we'll discuss in some depth in Chapter Nine, the relationship between the production of serotonin and melatonin is a close one, and the influence each substance has on our physical and psychological behavior is widespread.

What is melatonin's main function?

It now appears that the pineal gland and melatonin are the body's primary timekeepers—its clock and calendar—imparting information about the time of day, season of the year, and phase of life to the brain and throughout the body. In addition, melatonin is thought to help influence the internal orchestration of physiologic events and metabolic processes so that all of the body's systems work together, in coordination. Should this internal structure become disorganized in any way, the body becomes more susceptible to disease.

When do we produce melatonin?

Nicknamed "the chemical expression of darkness" by those who study the hormone, melatonin is produced almost exclusively at night or in a light-free environment. In fact, blood levels of melatonin are up to ten times greater at night than during the day. This high concentration of nocturnal melatonin led scientists to conclude that the production of this hormone signals to the rest of the body that it is time to sleep. Indeed, melatonin supplements have been used for decades to treat sleep-related problems, such as insomnia, sleep apnea, and jet lag.

In the morning, when we perceive that it is light, melatonin secretion ceases, which stimulates the production of other hormones and hence other body activities to begin. As we discuss in depth in Chapters Three and Eight, this orderly daily rhythm is of prime importance to our physical condition, intellectual capabilities, and emotional health.

In the animal kingdom, patterns of light and dark—and thus of melatonin secretion— also influence seasonal behaviors such as reproduction, hibernation, and migration. When daylight hours grow shorter during the autumn months, for instance, melatonin production in animals automatically increases, helping to make the almost constant sleep of hibernation possible. When daylight hours increase during the spring, the pineal gland secretes less melatonin, triggering a new pattern of physical activity.

The ways in which these seasonal patterns affect human behavior is under intense investigation. Some researchers believe that seasonal melatonin levels may help to explain a condition like Seasonal Affective Disorder (SAD), a depression that affects millions of men and women during the winter months when sunlight is scarce and nights are long (more on SAD and other psychological disorders in Chapter Nine). The tendency of most people to gain weight during the fall and winter every year may also be explained, at least in part, by the seasonal fluctuations of melatonin and other hormones.

In fact, a new science called chronobiology has emerged in recent years. Chronobiology explores the connection between the rhythms of nature—temperature fluctuations, weather systems, patterns of light and dark, among others—and the life cycle of men and women. We explore this emerging field further in Chapter Three.

Does everyone produce melatonin?

Yes, to some extent everyone produces melatonin. However, the amount of melatonin we produce depends upon our age and, to a lesser extent, upon our gender. In infants, for instance, the pineal gland is too small and underdeveloped to secrete much, if any, melatonin, which may be one reason that their sleep patterns are so unpredictable. Melatonin production appears to be at its greatest level during our teens and early adulthood.

Levels begin to drop off as we pass into our thirties and forties and, by age seventy or eighty, we secrete very little melatonin.

As for the influence of gender upon melatonin levels, recent studies indicate that women seem to be more sensitive to seasonal changes in light than men, and thus produce more melatonin in winter than in summer. Men, on the other hand, produce about the same amount of the hormone all year long. This fact may help to explain why women are more apt to develop dysthymia (low-grade depression) and to gain weight during the winter than their male counterparts. Our lifetime supply of the hormone, however, is about equal: Men and women begin to lose the capacity to secrete melatonin around the same age.

If our bodies produce melatonin, why should we take supplements?

For two reasons. First, our natural levels of this essential hormone decline because, for reasons not yet understood, the pineal gland begins to shrink as we age and thus cannot secrete as much as it could when we were younger. Second, the modern world in which we live and the hectic lifestyles most of us lead tend to suppress the amount of natural melatonin in our bodies.

This suppression may occur in two ways: First, we live in a world nearly devoid of regular rhythms of light and dark. Round-the-clock artificial light and other visual stimulants, especially television, work to wreak havoc with our bodies' natural pattern of hormone production.

Second, harmful substances known as free radicals may destroy both melatonin itself and the cells of the pineal gland, thereby decreasing the amount of melatonin in our bloodstreams.

In fact, a number of environmental and dietary factors that may have a negative impact on melatonin production have been identified. Alcohol and caffeine consumption, exposure to radiation and electromagnetic fields, sleep deprivation caused by overwork or night-shift employment, and a general resistance to natural rhythms all contribute to free-radical production and thus the need many us have for extra melatonin. These factors are addressed further in Chapters Four and Six.

Does everyone need to take melatonin supplements?

Probably not. Most men and women under the age of forty produce enough natural melatonin to provide them with all of the hormone's benefits. Unless they wish to reset their body clocks after jet lag or unless they suffer from a sleep disorder like insomnia or delayed sleep disorder, people under the age of forty probably do not need to take melatonin supplements on a regular basis. Unless under a doctor's care and careful observation, women who wish to become pregnant probably should not take melatonin on a regular basis, as it may disrupt their menstrual cycles (more on that issue in Chapter Eleven).

Apart from these general recommendations, it should be noted that no serious side effects from taking melatonin have been observed in any population to date. Even when large doses of melatonin—far more than would be prescribed to anyone hoping to improve sleep or provide extra protection against disease—have been administered in long-term laboratory studies, the benefits of taking extra melatonin appear to far outweigh the only known side effects. These still relatively rare side effects include excess sleepiness during the day or, conversely, sleeplessness during the night.

Nevertheless, there still is much we don't know about melatonin and its widespread effects on the body. Therefore we encourage you to discuss using melatonin with your doctor before you begin to take supplements, and certainly before you take significantly more than is recommended by most experts (about 5-to-10 milligrams per day).

Exactly what does melatonin do in the body?

Melatonin appears to affect the body in several different ways: as a potent master hormone, a powerful antioxidant, and a key component of the immune system. Let's examine these roles one by one:

Master hormone. Hormones are chemical triggers of body actions and reactions. Virtually every physiological process, from sleep to digestion to memory retrieval, is launched and carried out with help from these substances. Research emerging from laboratories around the world indicate that melatonin acts as a prime stimulator of hormonal activity. For instance, the blood level of melatonin appears to trigger the adrenal glands and go-

nads to increase or suppress the secretion of
male and female sex hormones; its role in inhibiting the production of estrogen is being
explored as a way to prevent or slow down
the development of certain cancers of the female reproductive system.

The presence or absence of melatonin also affects the production of pituitary-gland hormones,
including human-growth hormone. Human-
growth hormone regulates protein synthesis
(vital to muscle and bone strength) and energy
metabolism, among other essential functions.
Other important hormones secreted by the pituitary include oxytocin, which causes strong contractions of the uterus during pregnancy and
causes milk to flow from breasts. Research continues on the impact that melatonin may have on
other parts of the endocrine system.

Immune-system booster. Comprised of billions of blood cells and several hard-working
organs, the immune system is the body's primary defense organization. Its job is to protect
the body from invasion by harmful foreign
substances as well as to identify and destroy
errant or mutated human cells. As we discuss
further in Chapter Five, the presence of melatonin appears to increase the level of circulating immune-system cells, thereby bolstering
the body's ability to fight against diseases of
all kinds, from the common cold to cancer.

In animal trials and human tests, melatonin
stimulates the production of antibodies, the
first-line defense against infection. It restores
production of natural killer cells, a critical

part of the immune system and one that appears to decline with age.

Super antioxidant. According to current research, melatonin may be one of our most effective weapons against free radicals, substances that appear to be among the human body's most pervasive and damaging enemies. Free radicals are highly reactive molecules that can alter our DNA (the genetic code regulating cell growth and activity), damage proteins (the main building material for muscles, blood, skin, nails, and organs), and disrupt other bodily constituents. Free-radical damage has been linked to myriad age-related diseases, including atherosclerosis and cancer, as well as to the cosmetic effects of aging, such as the wrinkling of skin and graying of hair.

In the human body, the most damaging free radicals are derived from the chemical process by which oxygen is utilized inside the cells. Antioxidants are substances that render these free radicals harmless. By working to neutralize marauding free radicals, melatonin helps to prevent, or at least slow down, the steady and ultimately disease-producing erosion of healthy cells.

If melatonin is indeed as vital a substance as is suspected, its importance to healthy living cannot be underestimated. As a hormone, melatonin influences the aging process, reproductive cycle, sleep patterns, and a host of other integral physiological activities. By boosting the immune system, melatonin helps keep the body's innate and natural defense system alert and strong. And, as an antioxidant, melatonin limits the damage to organs and tissues caused by all-too-common substances on a molecular level.

How can melatonin have such a widespread influence on the body?

For two reasons. First, melatonin's ubiquitous presence throughout the body is partly due to its unique structure. A tiny molecule that is both water- and fat-soluble, melatonin can freely cross cell membranes and the blood-brain barrier. It can be found in the watery interior of cells and their protective perimeters, and is especially comfortable in the nucleus of the cell, protecting the genetic language encoded in the DNA from free-radical damage. Other antioxidants, like vitamins C and E, on the other hand, have much more limited access: Vitamin C occupies only the watery inner part of the cell, while vitamin E is confined to the fatty membranes.

Second, as discussed previously, melatonin works to trigger other hormones and neurotransmitters to carry out critical physiological functions. It is perhaps in this role—as an organizer and stimulator of other activities—that melatonin's greatest influence is expressed.

Is melatonin related to melanin, the substance that affects skin and hair color?

A study conducted in 1994 at the University of Colorado Health Sciences Center confirmed research showing no link between melatonin and skin color—at least not in humans and other warm-blooded mammals. In cold-blood reptiles, however, there is considerable evidence that melatonin may be involved in the species' ability to rapidly change skin color when stimulated to do so by changes in light exposure. Furthermore, melatonin levels appear to have no effect on the development of melanoma, skin tumors comprised of melanin cells.

Do I need to see a doctor to find out if I'm producing enough melatonin on my own or if I should take a supplement?

Generally speaking, no. Your own body should tell you when your natural supply of melatonin is dwindling: Your sleep patterns become disrupted, the first few gray hairs begin to sprout, weight seems to come on—and stay on—more readily, colds and other infections develop more quickly than before, and you've celebrated at least your fortieth birthday.

At the same time, it might be helpful for you to ask your doctor to perform a simple blood test to measure your melatonin levels, as well as discuss taking melatonin. Just because you have—or have not—reached a certain age, your melatonin levels might need some adjustment. If you've led a healthy lifestyle, one in which your exposure to free radicals has been limited, your supply of antioxidants rich, and your sleep patterns regular, you may have enough melatonin in your system no matter your age. On the other hand, someone in their late twenties who smokes cigarettes, drinks too much, and has a poor diet depletes his or her supply of melatonin more rapidly than healthier peers.

Remember, melatonin supplements are designed to restore a healthy supply of the hormone to your body, not to create an artificially high level in the bloodstream. In fact, because melatonin is a powerful stimulant of the reproductive system, too much melatonin given to a child or young adult may directly affect sexual development and reproductive health. (We'll talk more about the right way to take melatonin in Chapter Seven.) If you are unsure whether or not melatonin is right for you at this point in your life, talk to a physician.

When was the pineal gland first identified?

The history of this tiny gland is a long one. In the sixteenth century, French philosopher René Descartes referred to the pineal gland as the "seat of the soul," suggesting that this unpaired brain structure would serve as the ideal position from which the soul could exercise its effects on the body. This theory influenced future philosophers to associate the pineal gland with sin and physicians of the same period to associate the gland with mental illness.

It wasn't until the late nineteenth century that an understanding of the true role of the gland began to develop. In 1898, a Swiss scientist, after discovering a tumor on the pineal gland of a four-year-old boy who had gone into premature puberty, postulated that the pineal influenced the sexual maturation process, probably by inhibiting release of sex hormones in some way. More than sixty years later, in 1959, the first proof that the pineal did indeed exert a strong influence on human physiology came about when the gland's primary secretion, melatonin, was isolated and identified as a hormone.

Finally, during the 1980s, melatonin's role in the body became the subject of intense study. Scientists all over the world were surprised by the number of organs and physiological processes that appeared to be regulated by this substance. In 1985, researchers in the United States started to investigate whether oral doses of melatonin might be able to "trick" the body into thinking that it was nighttime, thereby making it possible to shift the human body clock backward or forward. These early studies proved that the hormone did indeed promote sleep much earlier than usual: When melatonin supplements were given to a group of insomniacs, for instance, they were able to fall asleep earlier and sleep more deeply than before.

Another study, performed at about the same time by a group of Italian researchers, centered on the effects of melatonin on a group of mice. Ten mice were given a small dose of melatonin every night, while ten others were denied it. Five months into the study, the researchers were astonished to see that the mice drinking plain water showed remarkable signs of aging: they had lost weight, slowed down their activity levels, and had patchy, drab fur. Those who drank water laced with melatonin, on the other hand, appeared and behaved much younger. In the next few weeks, the control mice began to die while the treatment group continued to thrive. In fact, the mean survival time of the untreated mice was 752 days compared to 931 days for the treated mice, a remarkable 20 percent increase in life span. And—best of all—their youthful appearance and vitality remained intact almost until the moment they died. The results of this study were confirmed by later ones in which the pineal glands of young mice were transplanted into the brains of older mice. Again, the test animals lived in good health far beyond their normal span.

Why would melatonin keep the rodents looking and behaving younger than their age?

No one knows for sure. Since melatonin appears to have a profound effect on several different systems of the body, it is likely that the answer will be a compound one. Its role as an antioxidant might be protecting skin and fur, as well as brain cells, from becoming damaged by free radicals, thus helping the mice to retain healthy coats and stay alert and vital. Boosting the immune system may also help the body fight against infectious agents and potentially cancer-causing cell mutations, which would greatly extend the life span. Merely by keeping the body in a regular pattern of sleep and wakefulness through the seasons of the year, and the years of life, melatonin may produce a host of health-enhancing effects as yet unknown.

There is one other possibility, one that we discuss in more depth in Chapter Two. Melatonin may protect against a built-in "aging clock" that is triggered to run down and give out at a genetically programmed time. When melatonin levels drop, that clock begins to tick, louder and stronger, with every passing year. If, on the other hand, we replace what is lost, it may be possible to turn the clock back or at least slow down its pace considerably.

What other studies are being conducted on melatonin?

In the past, melatonin's role as a sleep aid for jet-lag sufferers and insomniacs has come under the most scrutiny. Today, the scope of inquiry continues to widen:

- A group of scientists in the Netherlands has started clinical trials to test a contraceptive pill containing melatonin, which along with preventing pregnancy would decrease the risk of breast cancer.

- Studies involving the use of melatonin as a chemotherapeutic agent to treat brain, breast, lung, and other cancers have been launched at the Mary Imogene Bassett Hospital in Cooperstown, New York, and at research centers in Italy, France, and Spain.

- At the Oregon Health Sciences University, the University of Texas Health Science Center, and elsewhere, scientists continue to explore the relationship between melatonin and psycho-neurological disorders such as depression, Alzheimer's disease, schizophrenia, and bipolar disorder.

- At the Biancalana-Masera Foundation for the aged in Italy, University of Texas Health Center, and other research centers, the antioxidant role of melatonin as it applies to heart disease, arthritis, and other degenerative conditions remains under investigation.

Why are we just now hearing about melatonin? Is it just another fad?

The first question is simple to answer: We needed advanced technology to first identify, then isolate and extract, melatonin for study. Humans produce melatonin in mere picograms—one trillionth of a gram—and chemical reactions, like the oxidation of cells, take place in mere nanoseconds—one billionth of a second. Only by using recent medical and research tools could scientists begin to accurately assess melatonin's potential.

Whether or not melatonin is just another medical "phenomenon of the week" remains to be seen. However, the evidence that melatonin has profound and widespread effects on the body is overwhelming and mounting every day. And one can derive some reassurance that these studies are not prompted or promoted by pharmaceutical companies seeking to make a profit on an expensive prescription medication. Melatonin is a natural, organic substance for which there is no patent or ownership, which is why it is still inexpensive and widely available without prescription.

In this book, we attempt to provide you with all the information you need to decide—perhaps with help and advice from your doctor—whether or not taking melatonin supplements is right for you. At the same time, we hope to share with you some insight into the laboratory of minor and major miracles that is the human body, and to stimulate your interest in staying young and healthy for as long as possible.

• 2 •

The Biology of Aging

Why do we grow old?

On the surface, this question might seem more appropriate for philosophers to answer than physicians or scientists. Quite apart from its far-reaching moral and spiritual aspects, however, this question can be considered from a strictly biological perspective as well.

According to an old and widely accepted theory, we age and finally die in order to make room on this planet for the next generation of human beings to live and thrive. Should the mortality rate fall—if fewer people die than are born—the Earth could become overpopulated (something some scientists believe has already occurred), which would strain natural resources and thus put the entire ecosystem and all its life forms at risk.

This same general process takes place on a molecular level as well: When certain individual cells within an organism wither and perish, they are replaced by new cells able to function with vitality and health. In fact, each cell has information about its life cycle encoded within its DNA, the genetic blueprint found in the cell nucleus. When cells do not mature, reproduce, and then die according to this plan, the overall health of the organism may be comprised.

An example of such a disruption in a cell's life cycle is the disease we know of as cancer. For reasons not yet fully understood, cancer cells no longer have, or no longer heed, correct genetic messages about reproduction and death. They grow indiscriminately, using up nutrients meant to nourish healthy cells, which then shrivel and die before their time. If left unchecked, cancer cells grow and spread until the organism as a whole is unable to function.

Biologically speaking, then, aging and death are essential and quite natural aspects of all living things. And yet, because of our very "humanness"—the deep emotional and intellectual ties that bind us so intimately to earth and to each other—we continue to look for ways to circumvent this seemingly inevitable process. And the more we learn about the human body and its aging cycle on a molecular level, the more possible such a goal appears to become.

What happens to make the body age?

In essence, aging and death occur when cells within the body die or malfunction and are not replaced or repaired as rapidly as they should be. Eventually, the system or organ affected by cell death or mutation will no longer be able to operate properly. And, because human physiology is so interdependent, disruption in one part of the body often has widespread effects.

The most commonly fatal diseases of aging—heart disease and cancer—as well as age-related chronic conditions such as arthritis and senile dementia, all are related to what appears to be an inevitable loss of healthy cells and the chain reaction of damage that often results. Until medical science can find a way to halt this decline, our bodies are designed to fail in one way or another as we age.

Do researchers know what sets this process in motion?

Exactly how and why cell death occurs remains the subject of intense interest and study. In fact, gerontologist Zhores Medvedev identified and reviewed more than 300 different theories of aging in an article he wrote in 1990 for Biological Review—and all of them appear to have some merit. For the purposes of this discussion, we can narrow down the scope to four of the most generally accepted hypotheses:

Programmed cell death. Some scientists ascribe to the theory that every organism has an innate, species-specific life span. That's why most dogs have a life span of about twelve years, fruit flies approximately twelve months, and human beings about seventy-five years, to cite just a few examples. According to this theory, death, like all other physiologic activities, is genetically programmed into an organism's every cell. Exactly which and how many genes are directly involved in regulating human aging is still unknown, but some geneticists estimate the number to be about 200.

Free-radical damage. Another theory about aging centers on substances called free radicals. A free radical is a molecule that possesses an unpaired electron, one which is constantly attempting to become whole by robbing components from healthy cells. Unfortunately, this damages healthy cells, sometimes beyond repair. The body is thought to become more vulnerable to free radicals with advancing age; we produce more free radicals *and* are less able to defend ourselves against them. Scientists believe that the damage done to enzymes, proteins, cell membranes, and DNA by these harmful substances may lead to the development of several age-related diseases, such as atherosclerosis, cancer, Alzheimer's disease, and others.

Free-radical damage also is linked to some of the more cosmetic impacts of aging. Dermatologists estimate that as much as 70 percent of age-related skin damage comes from exposure to free-radical-rich ultraviolet rays from the sun. (Free radicals are further covered in Chapter Four.)

DNA damage. Some scientists postulate that the symptoms and side effects of the aging process could occur as a result of a series of mistakes made in the genetic blueprint encoded in every cell's DNA. As a cell ages, it becomes less accurate in its reproductive process for a variety of reasons, including an age-related increased vulnerability to free-radical damage as well as a decreased ability to repair itself. When genetic errors accumulate, the tissue the cells comprise becomes damaged, unable to function properly. Depending on what part of the body is involved, this degeneration of cells could lead to any of a number of age-related conditions.

Hormonal disruption and failure. Another theory about the cause of aging centers on the endocrine system. Indeed, some gerontologists believe there is an aging clock somewhere in the brain—probably in the hypothalamus or the pineal gland—which is directly related to hormonal secretion.

As we age, the amount and type of hormones our body secretes changes dramatically. This alteration in hormone secretion eventually results in a body-wide imbalance that affects the health of our immune system, metabolism, and reproductive ability. We therefore become ever more susceptible to disease and disability, as well as to the kind of cosmetic changes associated with aging—the wrinkling of skin, loss of muscle tone, weight gain, and graying of hair, to name a few.

So which theory explains why older people tend to get sick more often, and with more chronic and ultimately fatal illnesses, than young people?

It is likely that aspects of each of these theories, and others, are involved in the aging process. It is clear, for instance, that men and women have a rather fixed amount of time to live (no one has survived beyond the age of 120 and most people die at about seventy-five)—a duration that no doubt is genetically programmed in some way.

At the same time, free-radical damage has been linked to the development of several age-related diseases. Parkinson's disease, for instance, involves the gradual but inexorable death of certain brain cells, and most researchers point to free-radical damage as a likely cause. Parkinson's disease tends to develop in old age after a lifetime of exposure to free radicals and the chemical warfare they wage on the body and the brain.

More and more, however, scientists are considering the possibility that the endocrine system—specifically the hypothalamus and/or its close neighbor the pineal gland—might lie at the center of the mystery. Its effect on the body is so widespread, and its involvement in growth and maturation throughout life so intimate, that many people believe its role in the aging process is equally pivotal.

What role does the pineal gland play in our life cycle?

Research reveals that the pineal gland may well be the "aging clock" scientists have been searching for. The pineal gland appears to act as the body's timekeeper by keeping the body in sync with the most constant environmental cue we have: the light-dark cycle.

It is the pineal's job to announce to the rest of the body that it is dawn or dusk, time for the body to be awake and alert, or time to prepare for bed and a rejuvenating sleep. This crucial signal sets complex processes into motion, a cycle that is designed to remain relatively regular and balanced. As we explore further in Chapter Three, this so-called circadian rhythm lies at the heart of the state of internal balance and harmony we know of as health. When it becomes disrupted over a long period of time, there may be serious physical and psychological consequences.

At the same time, the pineal gland also appears to act as the body's pacemaker, a kind of "activities director" for the human life cycle. Scientists believe that the pineal gland, through its major product, melatonin, triggers the start of puberty and regulates reproductive life. When the pineal gland stops giving out its melatonin-directed signals, we grow old because our bodies are no longer able to operate with efficiency or with internal synchronicity.

Why do researchers call melatonin the master hormone?

As the pineal gland's major product, melatonin appears to directly affect the production and subsequent action of nearly every other hormone in the body. Researchers believe that melatonin has a great influence on the sexual maturation process by regulating the production of sex hormones. Children born with pineal glands, or who develop pineal tumors, for instance, tend to enter puberty prematurely. As mentioned in Chapter One, it was an 1898 Swiss physician who first linked the pineal gland with sexual development when he treated a boy with a pineal tumor who had gone into puberty at the age of four. Despite his age, this young boy had developed some secondary sex characteristics, including growth of pubic hair, enlargement of the testes and penis, and the deepening of his voice.

In addition, melatonin works in sync with serotonin, a powerful neurotransmitter from which it is derived. Serotonin is involved in several central physiological processes, including pain perception, temperature and blood-pressure regulation, and several neuropsychological functions such as appetite, memory, and mood. Like melatonin, serotonin levels influence a myriad of endocrine activities, including those performed by the hypothalamus and pituitary gland.

Generally speaking, the two related substances are not active in the body at the same time—melatonin rules at night, serotonin in the daytime. Although both tend to moderate endocrine functions, serotonin may also have a negative effect on the cardiovascular system if its levels are too high in the bloodstream. It has been known to cause blood cells to stick together and blood vessels to narrow, among other problems. And, unlike melatonin, serotonin levels in the body do not decrease as we age, but instead increase in relation to other hormones and neurotransmitters. Some gerontologists believe that this age-related imbalance between serotonin and melatonin may play as important a role in the aging process as the lack of melatonin itself, particularly in relation to heart disease. Without melatonin to act as a free-radical scavenger during the night, more damage may occur to blood vessels, thus stimulating the release of more serotonin.

How does the amount of melatonin change as we age?

We start out producing very little melatonin as babies: Studies show that rhythmic melatonin excretion does not begin until an infant is nine to twelve weeks old. By the time the baby is twenty-four weeks, total melatonin excretion is still only about 25 percent of adult levels. Slowly but steadily throughout childhood, melatonin excretion increases (as the pineal gland matures) and becomes more regular—a happy occasion for most parents, since the baby finally settles into a standard sleep schedule. Melatonin levels reach an all-time high during adolescence. Once full physical maturity has been reached, the pineal gland begins to shrink and melatonin levels slowly drop off.

The number of pineal gland cells appears to be genetically determined so that they decrease in number as we age. In addition, free radicals can damage pineal cells, causing the gland to deteriorate prematurely. In either case, the older we get, the less melatonin the pineal gland produces. This decline in hormonal output leads to fundamental changes throughout the body.

Does melatonin have an effect on menopause?

Melatonin is closely linked to the adrenal glands, which along with the ovaries, are primarily responsible for the secretion of estrogen and progesterone, the main female hormones. When melatonin levels drop as the pineal shrinks, the adrenal glands begin to slow down production of these hormones. Researchers believe the loss of melatonin may be the trigger that sets the process of menopause in motion.

Besides influencing fertility, what other role does estrogen play in the body?

Although the loss of sex hormones most directly affects the reproductive system, it also has an impact on a number of other physiological processes. For example, estrogen has been shown to have a positive effect on a woman's cardiovascular system, protecting her from the levels of heart disease suffered by her male peers. Postmenopausal women who do not replace estrogen, however, quickly develop the same kind of potentially fatal cardiovascular problems as do men.

At the same time, high levels of estrogen have been shown to influence the development of some cancers, such as endometrial cancer and a certain type of breast cancer. The risk of these cancers tends to rise according to a woman's age and to the number of years she has been producing estrogen. Recent studies, which are covered in depth in Chapters Ten and Eleven, have shown that the presence of melatonin offers a moderating effect on estrogen during a woman's youth and middle age, perhaps protecting cells of the uterus and breast from too much estrogen stimulation. At the same time that melatonin levels drop off as a woman ages, however, the risk of developing these cancers rises dramatically. The relationship between these two physiological events is still under investigation.

Indeed, the effects of estrogen on the female body are quite profound throughout one's life. In addition to its effects on the cardiovascular system, estrogen also appears to play a role in helping to keep skin supple and free of wrinkles, hair shiny and richly colored, bones strong, and muscles lithe—to say nothing of promoting a woman's sexuality and sex drive. Its loss helps to explain a host of age-related problems—both major and minor—from increased risk of heart disease and certain cancers to dry skin, osteoporosis, and loss of muscle tone. Chapter Eleven examines how melatonin supplements might be used to alleviate the symptoms and side effects of menopause when it does occur.

Do hormonal changes also affect men's health?

In men and women alike, reproductive health is directly related to both overall well-being and the rate at which health problems related to aging tend to progress. Although men do not experience as dramatic a change in hormonal fluctuations as do women, they are affected by the amount of testosterone and other male sex hormones circulating in the bloodstream.

Melatonin may play a similar role in moderating the effects of testosterone in men as it does with estrogen in women: When melatonin levels drop off as a man ages, the rate of prostate cancer and benign prostatic hypertrophy (overgrowth of prostate tissue due to testosterone) increases accordingly. More studies must be done in order to prove or disprove this hypothesis, however.

Do we lose any other hormones as we age?

It is important to stress that hormone levels increase and decrease every minute of the day in relation to our emotional, intellectual, and physical requirements. When we need food, for instance, certain substances are released to trigger the brain that we are hungry. When we first smell or taste food, other chemicals are released to prepare the stomach for the digestive process. Another chemical messenger lets the brain know when we are sated. For every physiological activity our bodies perform, similar coordinated—indeed elegant—orchestrations of chemical reactions take place.

As we get older, this highly complex system becomes imbalanced, either because an endocrine gland is lost (as is the case with melatonin) or because of another kind of breakdown in the body's ability to produce or use hormones properly. In the end, it is the balance and efficiency of the endocrine system and the processes regulated by it that matters most to our health and longevity. Keeping the body in balance by replacing hormones that are lost appears to be a key to delaying or slowing down the aging process.

How can melatonin be applied to the theories about aging?

Let's return to the four theories about aging outlined at the beginning of the chapter and see how melatonin affects each one:

Programmed cell death. It seems likely that the pineal gland itself is in some way genetically programmed to self-destruct as we age. Although scientists have yet to devise a way to reprogram DNA in the human brain, melatonin supplements allow us to replace what is lost and thus mitigate some of the ill effects of pineal decline.

Free-radical damage. When we lose melatonin, we lose one of our most powerful antioxidants. We are thus left more exposed to disease, disability, and discomfort. If we replace melatonin with supplements, we restore a powerful weapon to our arsenal against cellular injury by free radicals.

DNA damage. Melatonin helps to maintain the integrity of DNA in two ways. First, as discussed above, it acts as an antioxidant to protect DNA from free-radical damage. Second, preliminary research shows that melatonin somehow works to stimulate DNA's own repair mechanism. In effect, melatonin may help DNA correct its own errors before they can damage tissue.

Hormonal disruption and failure. It is as a master hormone that melatonin may most affect the aging process. We've already addressed its role in the reproductive system and the widespread effects changes in sex hormone levels can have throughout the body. In addition, the increase in serotonin relative to melatonin may also have age-related effects. As discussed above, too much serotonin in the bloodstream has been associated with an increased risk of atherosclerosis (a narrowing of blood vessels) and platelet aggregation (the tendency for certain blood cells to stick together, causing blood clots), both of which are serious—and all-too-common—age-related cardiovascular diseases. Replacing melatonin with supplements may help to moderate this negative serotonin influence.

What other factors influence how long we live?

Two rather fixed and uncontrollable factors have a great impact on how long individuals tend to live: our gender and our family history. Although the difference between male and female mortality rates has narrowed in recent years, there remains a gap of about five years. The reasons for this discrepancy involve a greater tendency among men to smoke cigarettes, work in jobs involving exposure to toxic chemicals, take physical risks (such as with dangerous sports or lifestyle choices), and experience high levels of emotional stress. As the gender gap within society continues to narrow, however, most epidemiologists believe that the mortality-rate variance will close up respectively.

What other ways might melatonin protect us from the aging process?

As discussed in Chapter One, melatonin appears to have a positive effect on our immune system, stimulating production of natural disease-fighting agents. When we lose melatonin, therefore, we become more vulnerable just when our body needs extra help to protect itself from the onslaught of age-related illnesses. Replacing melatonin may help to shore up our defenses at this crucial time in our lives.

In addition, melatonin's most immediate and well-known effects are those that involve sleep patterns, a subject covered in more depth in Chapters Three and Eight but which cannot be ignored in a discussion about aging and health. Sleep is as essential to health as food, water, or exercise. During sleep, our physical, emotional, and intellectual selves go through a period of rejuvenation and repair. Blood flow increases to the brain during certain sleep stages, bathing its cells in precious nutrients. The growth hormone, secreted from the pituitary gland (and also related to melatonin) during sleep, helps repair the damage done by the day's activity to cells throughout the body.

Finally, sleep helps to relax and relieve us from the physical and emotional stress of daily living. Although stress itself is not considered a disease from which we must recover, it can indeed aggravate or perhaps even provoke numerous conditions, including arthritis, atherosclerosis, cancer, diabetes, hypertension, and ulcers, among others. As you might be aware, the risk of developing these conditions tends to increase not only with stress but also with age. And melatonin might well be involved in this process as well.

How could stress act as an agent of aging and disease?

As discussed previously in this chapter, there is a close relationship between the pineal and the adrenal glands. In addition to stimulating production of the sex hormones, the adrenals also are involved in what is called the "fight-or-flight" response. When your body is threatened in any way, it mobilizes immediately, preparing you either to battle the impending danger or to flee from it. To do so, the adrenal glands release so-called stress hormones into the bloodstream that, in turn, cause various reactions to take place in the organs and tissues of the body.

Two of the most powerful stress hormones, norepinephrine and epinephrine, work to provide a fast and usually short-lived response to an immediate threat by stimulating the nervous system to raise the blood pressure, increasing the heart and metabolic rates, and making you breathe faster to provide more oxygen to your muscles. Later, other hormones, also excreted by the adrenal glands, are released to allow the body to continue fighting after the effects of the fight-or-flight response are over. These hormones, called corticoids, include cortisol and aldosterone.

Needless to say, the reactions induced during and after the fight-or-flight response are essential for our survival during times of great danger. However, problems occur when these powerful hormones and the reactions they stimulate continue over a long period of time due to perceived emotional or psychological pressure. Cortisol, for instance, is known to elevate blood sugar, increase platelet stickiness, and elevate serum cholesterol levels, all of which are risk factors for age-related cardiovascular disease and diabetes. Furthermore, chronic stress also has been shown to deplete the immune system, leaving us more at risk of developing illnesses of all kinds.

What does melatonin have to do with the stress response?

Generally speaking, melatonin appears to act as a corticoid antagonist; its presence tends to suppress the initial release of the hormones by inhibiting the adrenal glands. When we lose melatonin, potentially dangerous levels of corticoids are free to circulate throughout the body.

Again, however, it is not only the high level of corticoids that might influence disease development, it is also the disruption and disorganization throughout the body that is caused by any hormonal imbalance. Some scientists believe that abnormally high levels of corticoids at night (when they would normally be mitigated by the presence of melatonin) might help to explain some cases of senile dementia and other age-related disorders of mood and cognition. Replacing the melatonin that has been lost might help to reorganize this critical endocrine rhythm, thus resulting in widespread benefits to the mind and body.

Are there other ways to protect ourselves from the ravages of time?

In a famous study conducted at the University of Southern California School of Public Health during the 1980s, these seven healthy behaviors were found to have a significant influence on mortality rates:

1. consuming only moderate (or no) amounts of alcohol
2. eating breakfast on a regular basis
3. maintaining a healthy weight
4. avoiding fat-laden, sugary snacks
5. getting regular exercise
6. enjoying seven to eight hours of sleep a night
7. never smoking cigarettes

On average, men and women who followed these guidelines lived about nine years longer than those who had less healthy habits. More importantly, their quality of life at every age was significantly better than that of their peers. They suffered fewer chronic physical ailments and from less depression and other mood disorders.

It's important to keep these statistics in mind as you consider the role melatonin might play in your life: No matter how effective a longevity agent it might be, you will still bear the most responsibility for your own well-being through healthy eating, exercising, and other habits.

Is it possible that we will someday see human mortality rates increase, perhaps dramatically?

Think of it this way: During the Roman Empire, people on average lived only twenty-two years. In 1850, the average American died at forty-five, and by 1900, by forty-eight. Today, the average age at which Americans die is 75.8, and people over eighty-five constitute the fastest growing segment of the population. In fact, if current estimates are realized, there will be more than 200,000 men and women over the age of 100 living in the United States by the year 2020.

Add to this the remarkable research taking place in laboratories across the United States and around the world involving melatonin and other potential youth-enhancing treatments and philosophies and the possibility of expanding our life span—and improving the quality of life at every age—does not seem so far-fetched (more on longevity research in Chapter Twelve).

Could taking melatonin supplements keep me young forever?

Fortunately, the solution to the aging "problem" is not so simple. I say fortunately because there are so many ethical and environmental questions that society must answer before we put an end to the natural process of growing old and passing on.

On the other hand, there is every reason to suspect that taking melatonin supplements will help you stay healthier and feel more vital longer than might otherwise be possible—especially if you make a conscious effort to live well every day. If you exercise regularly, eat a proper diet, learn to relax and to avoid stress—as well as take melatonin supplements—you may be able to add several vigorous years to your life. Another important step to take is to learn to protect your body against damage from free radicals by both avoiding exposure to them as much as possible and by boosting your body's ability to neutralize them. This issue is explored further in Chapter Four.

In the meantime, let's take a look at one of the most studied aspects of melatonin: its effect on our sleep patterns and daily physiological rhythms.

• 3 •

The Inner Workings of the Body Clock

What is circadian rhythm?

From the Latin circa (about) diem (a day), the circadian rhythm is the twenty-four-hour cycle of light/dark, wakefulness/sleep to which most human physiologic processes are set. At regular intervals each day, the body tends to become hungry, tired, active, listless, energized. Body temperature, heart beat, blood pressure, hormone levels, and urine flow rise and fall in this relatively predictable, rhythmic pattern—a pattern initiated and governed by exposure to sunlight and darkness.

In the modern world, saturated with artificial light and loaded with constant stimulation, most of us attempt to rely completely on external signals to put our biological clocks in motion. We are not awakened at dawn by the sun, but earlier or later by an alarm clock. At night, the flickering of the television monitor keeps us up and stimulated long after natural nightfall might have triggered our bodies to prepare for sleep.

Nevertheless, the human animal retains a stubborn attachment to what seems a rather primitive code of behavior established by our most constant and eternal signal: the rise and fall of the sun. When we are forced to deviate from our natural pattern for any reason—because we travel across time zones, for example, or work the night shift—we often become physically and mentally disoriented until we can re-establish our connection to it. Long a subject of study by scientists interested in the physiology of sleep, the widespread importance of circadian rhythms to every aspect of our well-being has caught the attention of physicians, gerontologists, pharmaceutical companies, and millions of health-conscious men and women.

How does the brain know when it is light or dark?

Deep within the brain, inside an endocrine gland called the hypothalamus, lie two clusters of cells called the suprachiasmatic nuclei (SCN). The SCN—each of which are composed of more than 8,000 neurons—act as the body's circadian pacemaker. In mammals, the SCN appear to get their information from photoreceptors in the retina, which transmit signals about light and dark through the optic nerves to the hypothalamus. Once these messages enter the SCN, a series of physiological reactions takes place.

What happens after the light/dark signal reaches the SCN?

Interestingly enough, scientists are still unsure of exactly how the SCN spread the word about circadian rhythm to the rest of the body. It is known that the pathway from the retina through the optic nerves to the SCN extends further to reach the pineal gland, which lies adjacent to the hypothalamus above the brain stem.

Stimulated by the message it receives from the SCN, the pineal gland either secretes its main hormone, melatonin, or inhibits melatonin's release. As discussed in Chapter Two, the release of melatonin has far-reaching consequences on almost every system of the body, including the immune system, our free-radical scavenging capabilities, our reproductive cycles, and the regulation of powerful neurotransmitters that help to establish our psychological moods and intellectual applications.

Exactly what is the role of melatonin in the sleep/wake process?

Melatonin is both a sleep inducer and a product of sleep. Its production is stimulated by ambient darkness and suppressed by bright light, and its presence or absence in the body then helps to regulate other physiological rhythms. In experiments done with rodents, for instance, it was discovered that their eating, drinking, and sleeping patterns became disrupted when they were exposed to constant dim light—until and unless they were given an injection of melatonin at the same time every day. When that occurred, all of these functions become re-entrained to follow a regular schedule.

What happens to sleep patterns when we don't know if it's light or dark outside?

In today's world, most of us follow roughly the same pattern: Awake for about sixteen hours, asleep for about eight. When left to our own devices and separated from both natural and man-made imperatives, however, our bodies fall into a variety of different sleep/wake cycles. In some studies, people who lived for several weeks in a "time-free" room—isolated from all clocks or other hints of night or day—broke away from the twenty-four-hour clock and settled instead into a twenty-five to twenty-eight hour-a-day cycle. Rather than sleeping for eight hours straight through, the subjects of this study punctuated their days with one long rest period consisting of about five to seven hours of sleep, and a few short naps that added up to another two or three hours of sleep.

Another study showed a slight variation on that configuration: When kept in a time-free room for fourteen hours every night, a group of men slept about an hour longer than they normally did, but their sleep was spread out over about twelve hours. Early in the night, they slept for about four to five hours, spent several hours of quiet wakefulness in the middle of the night, then slept again for another four or five hours near morning.

What such patterns might mean to our health and well-being, however, remains a mystery. Only during the past few decades have medical techniques advanced enough for the physiology of sleep to be studied. And, despite the wealth of information that is now accumulating about its biochemistry and physiology, the precise nature and function of sleep is still largely unknown.

Is vision necessary for our internal clock to work?

Yes and no. The SCN and the parts of the brain that create images are supplied by different branches of the optic nerves so, technically, vision is not necessary for the brain to perceive that it is light or to tell the time. However, studies have shown that many totally blind people have free-running melatonin rhythms—rhythms that are not stimulated by how light or dark it is in the environment but by other as yet unknown information. And yet, although their cycles of hormone production, body temperature, and other physiological activities remain closely related to melatonin levels, they are able to sleep and wake according to a normal eight-hour/sixteen-hour schedule without associated fatigue or disorientation. Exactly how or why this is able to occur is still under investigation.

What is a zeitgeber?

One theory that explains how the blind organize their internal biological cycles—indeed, how we all are able to maintain our circadian rhythms despite a fundamental environmental mis-cue like an electric light—involves the idea of "zeitgeber." German for "time giver," a zeitgeber is any clue to the time of day presented to your body or your brain. Although sunlight and darkness remain the most obvious zeitgebers, we are surrounded by other hints, signs, and indications about the time of day—and our bodies appear relatively adept at following these clues as well. The smell of coffee brewing signals morning to many of us, the sound of the school bus chugging up the road and children laughing lets us know that it is midafternoon, the end of the late-night news frees up our minds and bodies to relax and snuggle down into sleep. In Chapter Eight, we'll show you ways to use zeitgebers of all kinds to re-entrain your circadian rhythm if it has been disrupted for any reason.

Why do we need to sleep?

The most widely accepted theory about sleep postulates that we fall into this state for two reasons: to conserve energy and to recuperate from the previous day's activities. Let's take them one by one.

First, we conserve energy when we sleep because our metabolic rate—the rate at which our bodies use energy to function—is reduced by at least 25 percent over daytime levels. Oxygen consumption, heart rate, and body temperature all decline during the first few hours of sleep and reach an all-time low about an hour before we wake up. In essence, then, sleep allows the body to maintain homeostasis—a relatively stable internal environment.

As for the recuperative and restorative powers of sleep, it appears that the whole body, including the central nervous system, needs to slow down in order to repair itself. We know that more than half of the total daily output of human growth hormone, a substance released by the pituitary and integral to growth in children and tissue repair in adults, is released during the first few hours of sleep. At the same time, cortisol and other corticoids, known to stimulate heart and respiration rates, fall to their lowest levels during sleep.

Many sleep experts, however, believe that it is the brain and not the body that benefits most from sleep. Indeed, studies have shown that sleep deprivation results in far more psychological than physical deficits—our concentration falters and our mood darkens far more quickly than our bodies experience any lasting physical impairments. In fact, people with insomnia or other sleep problems are more likely to develop psychiatric illnesses than their sleep-sated peers.

The truth is, however, sleep researchers still don't know with any certainty the specific biological functions of sleep. Indeed, people have been kept awake in experiments for as long as eleven days straight with no discernible physiological damage and only minor changes in circadian hormonal rhythms. On the other hand, no one can deny that a lack of sleep makes us at least *feel* bad—our mental performance and memory tend to suffer, we become irritable and/or anxious, and our physical reflexes falter, however temporarily. In the end, then, sleep is good for us, body, mind, and soul.

What happens during sleep?

Sleep is composed of two distinct physiological states, as different from each other in some ways as each one is from wakefulness. They are known as rapid eye movement (REM) and non-REM sleep and we pass through about four to six non-REM/REM sleep cycles every night. Let's look at each stage separately:

• Non-REM sleep consists of four different phases: Phase One is a light, drowsy sleep representing the transition from wakefulness to sleep and then, later, from sleep back to wakefulness. Phase Two is the first real stage of sleep, when your brain and body descend the long staircase into unconsciousness. Phases Three and Four are known collectively as "slow wave sleep" or "delta sleep." It is during this stage that body recovery is thought to occur. Blood flow is directed toward the muscles and organs of the body, and away from the brain, nourishing cells with nutrients and growth hormones. Furthermore, a study at the University of California School of Medicine connected slow-wave sleep to the regeneration of red blood cells.

- REM sleep, on the other hand, involves a dramatic increase of blood flow to the brain; estimates are that as much as a quarter of all blood circulating during REM sleep goes through the brain. Presumably, this increased blood flow is needed to support the many activities taking place in the brain during this period. First of all, we dream during REM sleep, and as we dream, our heart rate and blood pressure rises, metabolism speeds up, and our breathing gets faster and more irregular— all triggered by signals from the hypothalamus and other endocrine organs. Second, sleep researchers believe that short-and long-term memory are stored and other cognitive functions processed during REM sleep.

As people fall asleep, they progress through the non-REM stages and, then, about ninety minutes later, they have their first episode of REM sleep. As the night progresses, the episodes of non-REM sleep become shorter and those of REM sleep longer. Most slow-wave sleep occurs during the first third of the night, and most REM sleep during the last third.

How long does the average person sleep?

The majority of us (about 84 percent) sleep about 7.5 hours every night. But 15 percent of Americans get only 5.5 to 6.5 hours, while another 15 percent manage a full 8.5 hours.

About one in 100 people seem to thrive on only 5.5 hours, while another one in 100 seem to need 10.5 hours or more.

How do I know if I'm getting enough sleep?

A good rule of thumb is that if you wake up feeling rested and ready for action, you've slept enough. But because of the generally hectic pace of modern life, and the amount of external stimuli you probably receive on a day-to-day basis, you may no longer feel any connection to your physical body; you may not know how to listen to the signals about the need for rest and replenishment your brain might be sending you. That may be why stress-related diseases, including heart disease and certain cancers, are so prevalent. We talk more about sleep and how to make sure you're getting enough in Chapter Eight.

Is how long you sleep related to how tired you are or how long you've been awake?

The length of time a person sleeps is related more closely to body-temperature rhythms and bedtime than to how long the person has been awake, or even how exhausted he or she feels. In one study, even after being awake more than twenty hours, people free of time cues slept twice as long when they went to bed when their temperatures were at their highest (in the early evening) than when they were at their lowest (early in the morning). Again, this shows how closely tied we are to the biological circadian rhythm for cues about sleep and wakefulness.

How long can you stay up before you feel the effects of sleep deprivation?

When you stay up all night, fatigue increases from about 11 p.m until it reaches a peak at about 5 a.m. Assuming that you will be going to bed—or should be going to bed—your body temperature falls, melatonin is produced, and hormonal changes (such as a drop in epinephrine and cortisol) occur. Once you start to head into the morning hours, however, your body switches into its "awake" mode, with its temperature on the rise and epinephrine and cortisol surging. From that time forward, you're apt to feel better and more awake until the late afternoon, when you are likely to experience a sharp drop in attention levels and energy. Even if you feel exhausted, you will probably find it difficult to experience unbroken sleep starting at, say, 8 a.m. because your rhythm of body temperature and hormonal secretion are still following the natural light/dark circadian cycle.

Does how much sleep we need change as we get older?

Age is the most important factor affecting sleep. Infants sleep roughly twice as much as adults—as much as eighteen hours a day—and by age ten or so, most kids are down to about ten hours a night. Although some teens sleep more than their parents think possible, most develop a sleep pattern that approximates that of an adult.

The next dramatic shift appears in the elderly. By the time we reach our sixties and seventies, our sleep often becomes fragmented and disorganized. In fact, although older adults tend to spend about one hour *more* per night in bed, the biological rhythms that control sleep don't hold together as well. Dr. Charles Czeisler of Harvard's Brigham and Womens' Hospital and an expert in circadian rhythms has found through work at his lab that sleep cycles become shallower and more rapid in older people for a number of reasons. (In fact, the average sixty-year-old awakens more than twenty-two times a night, while a younger person in his or her twenties awakens just ten times.)

First, as we've discussed, the pineal gland shrinks as we age, inhibiting the release of sleep's most ardent promoter: melatonin. Responsible for setting the entire physiological stage for sleep, melatonin's loss makes it difficult for the body both to fall asleep in the first place and stay asleep once it does. Second, lifestyle changes that occur with aging also may have a significant impact on sleep patterns. Many older adults fail to get enough exercise and thus never really tire themselves out in a physical sense. Others develop low-grade depression and, though they feel lethargic, are too anxious and upset to sleep well. We'll offer hints on how to get a good night's sleep, no matter your age, in Chapter Eight.

Can we repair the damage done by lack of sleep?

A single night's sleep, one in which you let yourself sleep until your own body clock wakes is usually enough to for you to regain about 90 percent of the mental acuity you might have lost through sleep deprivation. A second full night of sleep restores the remaining 10 percent. In sleep experiments, people kept awake for three days sleep for about ten hours for two consecutive nights, and then, by the third night, return to their normal sleep patterns.

What happens to people who have to work the night shift? How do they work out their sleep patterns?

Millions of people around the world—about 20 million in North America alone—work at night. Because they commute home in the light, thereby signaling to their SCN that it is day and time for the body to be up and about, these workers often fail to adjust to their new schedules. If, on the other hand, they could somehow escape contact with light and instead make their way home in darkness, their bodies might be fooled into thinking that work time was daytime, no matter when it occurred. Another mistake made by many night-shift workers is trying to switch back into a daytime schedule during their weekends and vacations, thereby frustrating any attempts to set up a new cycle. Chapter Eight discusses light therapy and light-management techniques that have been used to entrain a new circadian rhythm in night workers, as well as show how melatonin can be used as a resetting tool.

Can melatonin help people with insomnia?

The causes of insomnia are complex and include dietary considerations (particularly caffeine, alcohol, excess carbohydrates and/or sugar), smoking, lack of exercise, and psychological problems, such as depression and anxiety disorders. Even more common than insomnia is a syndrome called delayed sleep-phase disorder, a specific form of insomnia in which people are unable to fall asleep at the desired clock time, but have little difficulty in falling asleep if bedtime is delayed for several hours. The duration of sleep is usually normal, but sometimes people with this syndrome experience daytime sleepiness and fatigue.

Under the age of forty, it probably isn't a lack of melatonin that's interfering with proper sleep patterns found with insomnia or delayed sleep-phase disorder, but melatonin supplements can nonetheless be used to help re-entrain an appropriate cycle. Chapters Six and Eight provide you with more information about treating sleep disorders.

Is jet lag related to melatonin depletion?

Not exactly. What jet lag involves is a desynchronization of the circadian rhythm. It usually is caused by traveling across several time zones within several hours, resulting in feelings of disorientation and fatigue. In fact, the symptoms and causes of jet lag are similar to problems that arise from working the night shift: Your body is telling you it's one time, while all the external zeitgebers are telling you it's much later or much earlier. Explored fully in Chapters Six and Eight, it is possible to use melatonin—usually along with light therapy—to re-set your internal circadian rhythm should it become disrupted by travel, work habits, or a bout with insomnia. And keep in mind that there are a host of other cures and solutions, ranging from getting regular exercise, to avoiding caffeine, to establishing rituals that prepare your body and mind to rest that can significantly improve the quality of sleep whether you decide to use melatonin supplements or not.

Besides triggering wake-sleep patterns, what other impact does the circadian cycle have on our bodies?

As we've discussed, hormone levels rise and fall in reliable patterns throughout the day, week, month, and year. The same is true for body temperature and other physiological activities. Indeed, it seems that almost every body function has its own window of opportunity in the biological cycle: Short-term memory, for instance, peaks in the morning, while the senses sharpen in the early evening. Studies show that sensory acuity is highest at 3 a.m., then falls rapidly to a low at 6 a.m., then rises to another peak between 5 and 7 p.m. This cycle is apparently related to the hormone cycle: When corticoids like cortisol are released, sensory acuity falls. And here are just a few of the ways that diseases and symptoms are affected by the circadian rhythm:

- Asthma attacks are 100 times more common during sleep than during waking hours.

- Heart attacks are twice as likely to happen between 8 and 10 a.m. than at 4 a.m. or 6 a.m. or 6 and 8 p.m.

- Women go into labor most often between 1:30 and 2:30 a.m. and least frequently around midday. Births between 2 and 4 p.m. are associated with increased probability of complications in both baby and mother.

- People are most allergic around 11 p.m. while antihistamine drugs have the greatest impact in the morning.

- Mood disorder symptoms peak in cycles as well: Studies have shown that most suicides occur during the late morning and early afternoon, while the risk of attempted suicide is greatest in the early evening.

Why do most heart attacks occur during the first few hours of the morning?

The exact mechanisms for circadian variations in cardiovascular disease remain unclear, although several factors might apply. Heart rate, platelet stickiness, as well as plasma epinephrine and norepinephrine levels, all peak in the morning hours after awakening when the fall of melatonin stimulates serotonin and corticoid release.

Interestingly enough, the risk of heart attack is greatest whenever your *body* thinks it's morning: If you arrive in a country where the local time is 6 p.m., but your body thinks it's 8 a.m., the risk that you'll have a heart attack at that time is just as great as if you were at home in your own bed.

What is chronobiology?

Chronobiology is the study of these biologic rhythms as they apply to disease and medicine. Circadian rhythms may dramatically alter the occurrence or severity of symptoms over the course of the day. Rhythms also may influence the way patients respond to diagnostic tests and procedures, and to drugs, surgery, and other treatment.

At research centers, chronobiologists learn to treat people more effectively by first mapping out these rhythms, then designing therapies to better match them. Franz Halberg, head of the chronobiology laboratories at the University of Minnesota, envisions a time when everyone will have a profile of their own of key body rhythms and be able to use them to better organize their activities and health care priorities.

What kind of medical treatments might be influenced by circadian rhythms?

The potency and toxicity of many drugs (including narcotics, asthma medications, aspirin, and anti-cancer drugs, among others) depend, to a large degree, on when they are taken. Here are just a few results of studies performed at various laboratories and research centers across the United States:

- Studies performed at the Hermann Center for Chronobiology and Chronotherapeutics at the University of Texas in Houston found that patients given anti-inflammatory drugs for rheumatoid arthritis in the evening were more likely to experience pain relief in the morning and suffer less gastric irritation. But patients with osteoarthritis, in which symptoms tend to be more severe during the afternoon or evening, required morning or midday dosing in order for pain medication to be effective.

- Oncologist William Hrushesky of the Stratton Veterans Association Medical College studied a group of eighty women with advanced ovarian cancer. He found that 50 percent of those who took adriamycin at 6 a.m. and cisplatin at 6 p.m. still were alive five years later, while only 11 percent of those taking the same doses of both chemotherapeutic drugs in reverse order lived that long.

- The same physician found that premenopausal women undergoing surgical resection for breast cancer fared better if operated on in the middle of their menstrual cycle, when estrogen levels are highest, than at other times.

- Aspirin, ibuprophen, and other nonsteroidal anti-inflammatory drugs appear to remain excellent pain killers whenever they are taken during the day. However, as Chapter Eight further examines, ibuprophen can inhibit the release of melatonin and thus disrupt, rather than enhance, sleep. Some doctors recommend, therefore, that aspirin be used instead of ibuprophen at night, unless there are medical reasons for someone to avoid aspirin.

The goal of chronotherapeutics—timing drug treatment with respect to the patient's individual body rhythms—is to optimize the therapeutic effect while controlling or reducing the adverse effects without altering the functioning of the drug in the body.

What is circaseptan rhythm?

Still the subject of a great deal of speculation, a circaseptan rhythm is a seven-day cycle in which the biologic processes of life, including disease symptoms and development, revolve. For example, a prominent scientist in this field, Dr. Erhard Haus, claims that transplant patients tend to have more rejection episodes seven, fourteen, twenty-one, and twenty-eight days after surgery, and medication given at certain times during this cycle stand a better chance of working—and with fewer side effects—than at others. As the study of chronobiology expands, more solid information about the circaseptan rhythm and its implications for the treatment of disease is sure to emerge.

What kinds of seasonal changes are related to melatonin and the circadian rhythm in general?

So far, most research regarding seasonal cycle has been done in animals. One study

showed that when ewes are injected with melatonin in the spring, they will begin to ovu-
late, because their bodies think that autumn,
with its longer nights and rutting rams has
arrived. In some rodents, melatonin triggers
seasonal changes to the pigment melanin,
changing its coat to white in the winter and
brown in the summer.

Do human bodies change in accordance to the season?

Unlike mammals in the animal kingdom,
most of us humans living in the modern, industrialized world have pretty much dis-
tanced ourselves from experiencing any
fundamental physical and even emotional
changes with the seasons. Nevertheless, we
are not completely free from natural influences. For instance, people who live in parts
of the world where light/dark patterns are
extreme, such as in the arctic, experience very
different melatonin secretion levels than those
with more standard exposure to sun. A 1993
study conducted by the Department of Arctic
Biology at the University of Tromso, Norway,
found that people exposed to twenty-hour
nights during the month of January had far
higher melatonin blood levels than they did
in June, when the sun was out for approximately fourteen to sixteen hours per day.

In Fairbanks, Alaska, researchers from the
Community Mental Health Services noticed a
similar pattern in a study they conducted in
1993, but they took it one step further. They
noted higher nighttime cortisol and daytime

melatonin during the winter months when compared to the normal pattern at lower altitudes. These findings imply possible underlying physiological causes for the high incidence of behavior disorders such as depression and alcoholism in Alaska and arctic regions in general.

A study of about 400 men and women conducted at Georgia State University in Atlanta showed that, on average, both men and women ate about 220 more calories a day in the fall (mostly in the form of carbohydrates) than in any other season and, even though they were eating more food, felt hungrier.

As Chapter One discusses, seasonal differences appear to be greater in women than in men. A recent study of 125 postmenopausal women showed significant increases in their bone and muscle mass after the summer-fall period and a significant decrease after the winter-spring period, while fat tissue decreased during the summer-fall and increased throughout the winter-spring. Exercise was the only thing that made a difference in their ability to maintain their weight.

In northern countries, in regions where a strong seasonal contrast in light/dark patterns exists, activity of the pituitary/ovarian axis and the conception rate are decreased during the dark winter months. In these areas, inversely, women experience a peak in conception rate during summer, leading to a maximum birth rate in the spring. While this also may be due to other factors as yet unknown, this information may prove to be particularly useful for in-vitro fertilization and infertility in general, a subject that Chapter Eleven examines.

How can melatonin be used in chronobiology?

The answer to that question remains the subject of great interest to scientists around the world. Now that it seems certain that the health of the organism depends to a large degree on a state of internal balance and rhythm—something that melatonin seems to control—more attention will be paid to treatments combining melatonin with light therapy, chemotherapy, etc.

At the same time, more research than ever is being done on another crucial aspect of physiology and one that interferes with health perhaps more than any other single environmental factor: free radicals. Chapter Four explores this important field.

• 4 •

Free Radicals and Disease

What is a free radical?

As discussed in previous chapters, free radicals are molecules that contain one or more unpaired electrons in their orbits. These unstable molecules, in an attempt to stabilize themselves, try to combine with nonradical cells in the body. By doing so, they often damage cell membranes as well as the internal structures of the nonradical cell, including the genetic material encoded in DNA.

There is growing evidence that the major "killer diseases" of the modern industrialized world, namely cardiovascular disease and cancer, are influenced by the presence of excess free radicals and the biochemical reactions they cause in the body. Later in the chapter, we'll discuss more fully how free radicals are involved in each of these diseases.

Where do free radicals come from?

Free radicals are produced inside the body. They also come into the body through the air we breathe. Every cellular process in the body creates free radicals as a consequence of using oxygen as an energy source. Immune-system function, metabolism, communication between cells, and even the production of collagen—the substance that forms connective tissue—all produce free radicals as a by-product of their processes. The richest source of free radicals, however, is the oxygen in the air we breathe. Every time we inhale a quart of air—the amount we breathe in about thirty minutes—we expose our cells to 1 billion free radicals.

Why is a free radical so dangerous to our health?

The damage done by a free radical goes beyond the first cell it attacks. Not only is that cell injured—its ability to reproduce and metabolize permanently impaired—but it, too, becomes a free radical, ready to ravage another healthy cell. This chain reaction may continue, deforming cell after cell after cell. If the resulting damage occurs in the immune system, you become more vulnerable to infections; when it happens to muscle tissue, muscle sprains and strains are more likely to occur. And when free radicals disrupt enzyme production vital for regulating biochemical reactions throughout the body, the stage is set for the premature aging of any number of systems and organs.

Are there different kinds of free radicals? Are some more damaging than others?

There are several types of free radicals, and they are different from each other in their biochemical makeup and their effects on the body. Hydroxyl is perhaps the most damaging to human cells. Although the original hydroxyl molecule has a short life span, it usually sets a chemical chain reaction—like the one described above—into motion.

Two much less reactive and potentially dangerous-free radicals are superoxide and nitric oxide. Some superoxide is generated as an accidental by-product of processes performed by catecholamines (like epinephrine and norepinephrine) and some constituents of mitochondria (the energy-producing structures in cells). Other superoxide is made deliberately. For instance, activated immune-system cells called phagocytes generate large amounts of superoxide as part of the mechanism by which they destroy foreign organisms. Nitric oxide is made as a by-product of a process within the tissue lining of blood vessels, as well as by phagocytes and brain cells.

What is an antioxidant?

The human body is a remarkably self-contained organism. It even has an elaborate built-in defense system against all kinds of enemies—including free radicals. Chapter Five explores the immune system, which attempts to destroy substances it identifies as "nonself" like bacteria, viruses, and even body cells that have mutated into cancer cells.

We also have vigorous anti-radical defenses called antioxidants—enzymes, vitamins, and minerals that mop up free radicals before they can do any harm. Some antioxidants are produced by the body itself and others are ingested. Superoxide dismutase, an enzyme found in mitochondria and cytosol (the liquid part of cells), is an example of an endogenous antioxidant—a substance the body makes itself. Superoxide dismutase disarms superoxide by converting it to hydrogen peroxide, which is then metabolized into water by yet another endogenous free radical called glutathione peroxidase.

In addition to these and other chemicals that act directly to protect the body against free-radical damage, the body also produces repair enzymes that help "clean up" after free-radical warfare. Substances called repair enzymes destroy proteins that have been mangled by free radicals, remove oxidized fatty acids from membranes, and restore free-radical damaged DNA.

Despite its complexity and elegance, our anti-free-radical system is often not strong enough to protect our bodies against the onslaught of unstable molecules that bombard us from the environment. Fortunately, we can reinforce our endogenous defenses by eating foods rich in antioxidants and/or taking antioxidant vitamin supplements. These possibilities are discussed later in this chapter.

Does melatonin play a role in the antioxidant defense system?

Most definitely, although researchers still are exploring its exact function. Recent studies, however, indicate that melatonin is one of the body's most potent and efficient free radical scavengers. Especially useful against the highly toxic hydroxyl radical, melatonin is able to provide on-site protection against oxidative damage to biomolecules within every part of the cell, from the fatty cell membrane to the DNA inside the nucleus.

Besides scavenging hydroxyl, melatonin also triggers other antioxidants into action, including glutathione peroxidase, which metabolizes hydrogen peroxide into water. Thus melatonin has at least two means to protect the cell from oxidative damage: It breaks down hydrogen peroxide to harmless water and, in the event that any hydrogen radicals are formed, melatonin is in a position to neutralize them before they can do any harm.

How does melatonin work as an antioxidant?

Once melatonin is produced in the pineal gland, its unique molecular structure allows it to readily pass through the membrane of the pineal cells and linings of the capillaries into the bloodstream. From there, melatonin readily escapes into every other bodily fluid, thus making it available to every cell in the body. Its high diffusability is essential to its scavenging capabilities because this feature allows it to enter at will all cells and every subcellular compartment, including the cell nucleus, the home of DNA.

The evidence of melatonin's value as an antioxidant continues to mount. Researchers at the University of Texas Health Center in San

Antonio have found that rats treated with melatonin and then injected with safrole—an unusually nasty free radical—sustained 40 to 99 percent less DNA damage than untreated rodents. Although the amounts of melatonin required to offer optimal protection would correspond to 10 to 40 milligrams for an average human—levels normally attained only at night and thus inappropriate for daytime scavenging—the potential of this natural hormone as an antioxidant is exciting.

What is the relationship between free radicals and heart disease?

Heart disease remains one of America's most pervasive and life-threatening health problems. Each year about 1.5 million Americans have heart attacks and 600,000 die from heart disease. Although many factors are involved in the development of heart disease, damage to the cardiovascular system by free radicals remains a significant risk for most Americans.

What causes heart disease?

Most all cases of heart disease are due to the progressive narrowing of the coronary arteries, which supply heart tissue with the blood it needs to survive. The narrowing is caused by atherosclerosis, a disease in which plaques made of fatty substances and blood clots collect on the inner wall of one or both arteries or, indeed, anywhere in the blood-vessel system.

The buildup of atherosclerotic plaque is

usually a gradual process; it may take decades before any symptoms of damage appear. The plaque gathers in response to damage to the inner wall of an artery. This damage can come from many sources: High blood pressure pushes against arterial walls with a greater than normal force and thus damages the lining. Toxic substances such as nicotine and asbestos irritate and damage the arterial lining. Hormones, during periods of high stress, often have an abrasive effect.

Does high cholesterol cause heart disease?

Research indicates that it is not the level of cholesterol in your blood, per se, that raises your risk for developing atherosclerosis. In fact, cholesterol is a lipid (fatlike substance) essential for a number of vital body processes, including nerve function, cell repair and reproduction, and the formation of various hormones, including estrogen and testosterone and the stress hormone cortisol. Before cholesterol can be considered harmful, it must be oxidized—changed into a free radical. Once it is oxidized, it acts as a lure, drawing other cells to it, precipitating a chain-reaction culminating in an artery-clogging plaque.

How is cholesterol oxidized?

Cholesterol travels through the bloodstream by combining with other lipids and certain proteins. When combined, these substances are called lipoproteins. One type of lipoprotein, called high-density lipoprotein (HDL), is beneficial to the body because it carries cholesterol away from the cells to the liver, where it is processed and eliminated from the body. HDL-cholesterol is known as the "good" cholesterol.

Another type of lipoprotein, however, is considered harmful to the body. Called low-density lipoprotein (LDL), this substance carries about two-thirds of circulating cholesterol to the cells. This is usually the "fat" we speak of when referring to the plaque that builds up and causes atherosclerosis.

Where do free radicals affect the development of atherosclerosis?

Current research indicates that LDL-cholesterol may become harmful only after it has been oxidized, or combined with oxygen—in essence becoming a free radical itself, a free radical called an oxysterol. Oxidized cholesterol enters the bloodstream either from processed foods, from ingested animal products, from environmental pollutants (particularly pesticides and chlorine), or from such internal stressors as infections and emotional stress.

Can antioxidants prevent the oxidation of cholesterol?

During the past decade or so, several studies have indicated that antioxidants, especially vitamin C, vitamin E, and beta-carotene (a precursor of vitamin A), are able to prevent, or at least slow down, the oxidation of cholesterol. During the early 1990s, experiments at the Center for Human Nutrition at the University of Texas Southwestern Medical Center in Dallas, showed that high doses of vitamin E—about 500 milligrams per day, or more than ten times the amount found in the diet— rendered cholesterol resistant to oxidation. While vitamin C and beta-carotene were not as effective in blocking the process, they, too, were helpful in hindering it.

Another major study, conducted by researchers at Harvard's Brigham & Women's Hospital in Boston, involved following the diet and health profiles of 87,000 women nurses over a ten-year period. Investigators found that the women whose vitamin-E consumption was in the upper 20 percent had a 35 percent lower risk of heart disease, even when all other risk factors, such as smoking, family history, and cholesterol levels were accounted for. Those whose beta-carotene consumption was in the upper 20 percent had a 22 percent lower risk of developing heart disease.

And, most recently, the Women's Health Study at Harvard University is testing whether 50 milligrams of beta-carotene every other day, alone or in combination with vitamin E and aspirin, can lower the risk of heart disease and cancer in women. Results are expected in 1996.

What other things can we do to protect ourselves from developing heart disease?

The following statistics about risk factors, published by the *New England Journal of Medicine* in 1992, sums up how much potential damage we can avert by complying with sensible lifestyle recommendations:

Quit smoking. Former smokers lower their risk by 50 to 70 percent compared with current smokers.

Exercise. Active people have a 45 percent lower risk than their sedentary peers.

Maintain ideal weight. Men and women who are at their ideal weight have a 35 to 55 percent lower risk compared with people who are 20 percent or more above their ideal weight.

Reduce serum cholesterol. For every 1 percent reduction in total serum cholesterol, people reduce their risk of heart disease by 2 to 3 percent. (Cholesterol levels drop an average of 10 percent with diet therapy and 20 percent with medication.)

Take one aspirin every other day. Men and women who take an aspirin every other day have a 33 percent lower risk compared to nonusers.

Other steps involve maintaining normal blood-sugar levels, consuming no more than one or two alcoholic drinks per day, and, for women, estrogen-replacement therapy after menopause (which lowers risk by 44 percent compared with non-users).

Why would aspirin protect against heart disease?

Aspirin blocks the body's production of protaglandins, potent hormonelike chemicals that aid in the formation of blood clots. Interestingly enough, some studies have shown that melatonin also helps block prostaglandin production, which is another way that taking melatonin might help prevent heart disease. If studies prove that theory out, it could mean that millions of people unable to take aspirin because they are allergic or because aspirin produces harmful side effects (like stomach irritation and intestinal bleeding) will have a safe and effective method of reducing their risk of heart disease.

Is the development or progression of cancer also affected by free radicals?

The cells in your body have an outer membrane made up of fatty material that protects against cancer-causing substances (carcinogens). When those walls weaken from oxidation—from free radical damage—carcinogens can easily enter the cell and disrupt its genetic code, in essence turning it into a cancer cell. A cancer cell then reproduces, abnormally and uncontrollably, passing on its mutation to each succeeding generation. Eventually, the entire organ where the original cell was damaged may be suffused with cancer cells that have formed a tumor. In some cases, cancer cells break off from the primary tumor and spread to another part of the body, a process known as metastasis.

Where do the free radicals that cause cancer come from?

Some researchers believe that cancer often begins when a body cell and its DNA are damaged by oxidants that come from everyday metabolism, from cigarette smoke, and even from chemicals the body itself produces to fight infection.

One of the most pervasive and potentially harmful sources of free radicals results from the emission of chlorofluorocarbons (CFCs) and similar substances that have caused a steady erosion of the ozone shield in our upper atmosphere. Without an ozone layer to protect us, ultraviolet rays can penetrate deep into the skin, which may account for more than 400,000 cases of skin cancer every year.

How can melatonin help prevent cancer?

As Chapter Ten discusses in depth, scientists believe that melatonin works on several levels to protect against cancer, including as a stimulator of the immune system and a hormonal regulator. For the purposes of this chapter, however, we want to re-emphasize the melatonin's role as one of the body's most potent antioxidants, able to protect cells from invasion by, and ultimate mutation by, free radicals.

Have studies been able to prove that antioxidants, like vitamins, minerals, and melatonin can protect against cancer?

Yes, several research studies have shown a definite correlation between high antioxidant diets and a lowered risk of cancer. In a five-year study of nearly 30,000 rural Chinese men and women conducted in the 1980s, for instance, researchers from the National Cancer Institute found that daily doses of beta-carotene (a precursor of vitamin A), vitamin E, and the micro-mineral selenium reduced cancer deaths by 13 percent.

Certain cancers seem more likely to be helped by antioxidants than others. Some studies have shown that cancers of the esophagus, oral cavity, stomach, pancreas, rectum, breast, cervix, and lung are those that appear to benefit most from antioxidant protection. Beta-carotene, for instance, appears to play a particularly important role in protecting women against the development of cervical cancer.

And research continues. The Physician's Health Study at Harvard is testing whether or not 50 milligrams of beta-carotene every other day can ward off cancer in men; the results should be available in 1996.

If I want to reduce my risk for heart disease, cancer, and other diseases caused by free-radical damage, what antioxidants do I need?

In terms of helping to protect your body against the onslaught of free radicals, there are four major antioxidant weapons available to you, both in foods and as supplements:

Beta-carotene (RDA 4,800 micrograms) is a plant pigment that gives carrots, apricots, and cantaloupe their orange color, but is also found in spinach and other leafy green vegetables. In the body, beta-carotene is actively converted into vitamin A, a powerful antioxidant. The apparent effects of beta-carotene are remarkable: One comprehensive study found that women who ate one carrot a day had a

68 percent less chance of having a stroke than those who ate one a month. To give you an idea of what it takes to fulfill your RDA, here are some food values: one carrot has 12,152 micrograms; half a cantaloupe contains 5,165 micrograms; and two cups of raw spinach 4,512 micrograms of beta-carotene.

Vitamin C (RDA 60 milligrams) is perhaps the most well-known and highly touted antioxidant. It is believed that it helps prevent the formation of oxysterols and protect the heart and vessels against free-radical damage by helping in the synthesis of collagen. Studies have shown that it may enhance the immune system, offering protection against the development of cancer and a host of other conditions, including the common cold. It's easy to meet your RDA requirements—one orange contains 124 milligrams of vitamin C; half a cantaloupe provides 113 milligrams, and one cup cooked broccoli, 98 milligrams—but the amount needed to provide antioxidant, anticancer benefits is still under investigation.

Vitamin E (RDA 8 milligrams), another powerful antioxidant, has the added benefit of being fat-soluble and thus able to prevent abnormal blood-clot formation and help repair free-radical damage to blood-vessel linings. In fact, a study funded by the World Health Organization showed that too little vitamin E in the body proved to be a greater risk factor for heart disease than either high blood pressure or high cholesterol levels in sixteen European study populations. Because the food sources of vitamin E—including vegetable oils and nuts—tend to high levels of fat, some people prefer to get their daily dose from supplements. There are, however, some fairly low-fat foods rich in this essential nutrient: one ounce fortified cereal provides 6 milligrams of vitamin E, one ounce dried almonds, 7 milligrams, and one mango, 2 milligrams.

Selenium (RDA 55 micrograms) is a trace micro-mineral, and scientists have only just recently begun to realize its importance as a potential disease-fighter. It is known to interact with vitamin E to prevent the breakdown of fats and body chemicals that could otherwise form free radicals. The best sources of selenium are fish and shellfish, followed by beef, chicken, whole grains, eggs, and garlic. High selenium levels also can be found in mushrooms, tomatoes, and radishes.

Is it better to get antioxidants from supplements or foods?

Research suggests that supplementing your diet with antioxidants—whether in whole foods or through vitamin and mineral supplements—can help to reduce your risk of free-radical damage. (This is especially true for smokers, who need an extra supply of antioxidants to fight the free radicals formed by tobacco use.) However, scientists still are unsure of exactly how much of these vitamins and minerals we need to take before protection from free radicals is assured—or, more importantly, how much will cause toxic reactions.

For that reason, most nutritionists would certainly encourage you to try to get all you need from your diet and, before taking supplements, discuss your nutritional needs with a physician. Generally speaking, it makes more sense to eat healthy foods and avoid exposure to toxins than to rely on a pill for protection. By doing so, you also stand a greater chance of providing your body with the raw material it needs, through the diet, to build and rebuild blood cells, muscle tissue, enzymes, hormones, neurotransmitters, and other body components. Of primary importance is a strong and healthy immune system, which is the subject of our next chapter.

• 5 •

Melatonin:
An Immune-System Booster

What is immunity?

The word immunity comes from the Latin
word *immunitas*, which in ancient Rome
meant the release of an individual from an
obligation to serve the state. Today, we also
use this word in a similar way. For instance,
when a known criminal testifies in court in
exchange for his or her own freedom, we say
they are "immune" from prosecution. To be
immune from a disease means that you are,
in a way, exempt from getting it. Your body
has specific mechanisms to protect you from
it.

Immunity from a disease develops when a
foreign organism or substance, called an antigen, enters the body and is recognized by certain blood cells. This recognition triggers
other blood cells into action, which either at-

tack the antigen directly or produce special proteins that neutralize it in other ways.

A strong and vigorous immune system is integral to the maintenance of health, but we all too often fail to give this essential part of our body the attention it deserves. As this chapter discusses, many of the lifestyle choices we make, and the environmental hazards that surround us, deplete the very cells meant to protect us against disease and disability. The loss of the hormone melatonin may be one reason why age-related diseases are allowed to take hold.

What organs and cells make up the immune system?

Although the strict parameters of the immune system are described below, it should be noted first that the human body has many ways of protecting itself from being invaded by potentially harmful substances. First, we have physical barriers that stop microbes, such as viruses, bacteria, protozoa, and fungi, before they can enter the body. Intact skin, for instance, is very difficult for most pathogens (disease-causing agents) to penetrate. Second, our body itself produces many substances that destroy foreign invaders quickly and efficiently. The fatty acids of the skin and an enzyme called lysosome, which is found in saliva, tears, and other body secretions, are such nonspecific defenses.

Our immune system is the main line of defense against pathogens virulent or lucky enough to bypass the body's protective devices. The human immune system has two components: a fixed compartment of organs and tissues and a circulating compartment consisting of a fluid called lymph and billions of circulating cells and molecules. Let's take each one separately:

The Organs

- Thymus (a gland located at the base of the throat behind the breast bone).
- Bone marrow (the soft, fatty tissue on the inside of bones).
- Lymph nodes (pockets of tissue located in the mouth, neck, lower arm, armpit, and groin).
- Lymphatic vessels (a system of ducts that collect fluid from the body's tissues, deliver it to the filtering lymph node, and transport it to the heart, where it rejoins the body's main circulatory system).
- Spleen (located in the abdominal cavity near the stomach).

The Lymph

- Lymph (a colorless liquid similar to blood but containing no red blood cells or platelets and which carries lymphocytes through the body).
- Leukocytes (another term for white blood cells, which are involved in protecting the body against foreign substances and in the production of antibodies).
- Lymphocytes (white blood cells responsible for the immune response; your body con-

tains one trillion lymphocytes, comprising about two pounds of body weight).

How do immune-system cells recognize substances as potentially harmful?

The immune system's special characteristic is the ability to recognize other cells in the body. It can tell the difference between harmful microbes, cancerous cells, and the body's own healthy cells. Put simply, it's as if every cell and microbe wears a uniform and the patrolling guards—the lymphocytes—are able to distinguish one uniform from another. Every different kind of cell wears a different uniform, and each must be responded to in particular, specific ways during the immune process.

When a cell provokes a response from the immune system, that is, when lymphocytes recognize an enemy uniform, an immune-system response is provoked. Transplanted tissues and organs, and sometimes even our own cells that have become cancer cells, also may be recognized as "non self," triggering an immune response.

Are there different kinds of lymphocytes?

Yes, there are a variety of immune-system cell types, each with its own set of responsibilities. Natural-killer cells, for instance, are large lymphocytes that can destroy diverse microbes on sight, as well as play a role in absorbing cancer cells. Phagocytes and macrophages, which originate in the bone marrow, are designed to ingest and digest foreign particles including some viruses and bacteria.

The division of labor in the immune system is further delineated. There are two kinds of antigen-specific immune responses, closely related and in some cases dependent upon one another. As their name implies, these responses are triggered by specific antigens—cells with specific uniforms recognized by lymphocytes.

Humoral immunity involves the production of protein molecules each time a new antigen is recognized. These molecules are called antibodies. The type of lymphocyte directly responsible for antibody formation is called the B cell. B cells are first produced in the bone marrow and have molecules on their surface membranes that correspond to a certain kind of antibody. These B-cells circulate in the body until they come into contact with an antigen that corresponds to its antibody structure. The antigen then locks onto the B cell, which provokes an immune response. The B-cell rapidly and repeatedly divides, creating hundreds of new cells that release antibodies in massive amounts.

Antibodies are antigen-specific, able to react only with the antigen that causes each to be produced. B cells also produce memory cells, cells stored in the lymph that have the ability to recognize the specific antigen that provoked their production. Should this antigen be reintroduced into the body, memory cells quickly divide and release appropriate antibodies immediately.

What are T cells?

T cells are lymphocytes that perform the other kind of immune-system response called cell-mediated immunity. T cells also are produced in the bone marrow but, unlike B-cells, make another stop in the thymus. The thymus takes immature lymphocytes and processes them into T cells (thymus-derived cells). T cells also have molecular codes on their surfaces that correspond to specific antigens. When T cells recognize and bond to antigens, cell-mediated immunity occurs. Some T cells—appropriately called TK for T-killer cells—are sensitized against particular antigens, releasing a lethal poison immediately upon contact.

The rest of the T cells are divided into two major subsets: T-helper cells and T-suppressor cells. These cells work together with other immune-system cells to create the immune response. T-helper cells, as their name implies, call macrophages and TK cells into action and stimulate B cells into antibody production. T-helper cells are the "on switch" for the fight against many microbial infections.

T-suppressor cells are the "off switch." When the crisis is over and the invading microbe has been dealt with, T-suppressor cells signal to other lymphocytes that the danger is over. Macrophages move away, TK cells stop reproducing, and B cells halt their production of antibodies.

T cells communicate these messages to other lymphocytes by releasing enzymes, peptides, and proteins, and by other means as yet unknown. What is known, however, is that when either the cell-mediated or humoral branch of the immune system malfunctions or is depleted, we become vastly more vulnerable to disease.

What are allergies and autoimmune diseases?

Although quite different in their causes and their effects, both of these conditions can be considered to be overreactions of the immune system.

In most cases and for most people, the immune system works efficiently to protect the body from harmful foreign invaders. With allergies, however, the immune system "misreads" the signals and responds to substances that are actually benign. Such reactions involve an interaction between a specific foreign substance—pollen, for instance, or cat dander—called an allergen and a specific antibody. When an antibody attacks an allergen, it does so by releasing a substance called histamine, a body chemical that can act as an irritating stimulant, and other chemicals into the tissue. These chemicals act to produce symptoms common to what we know of as the allergic response: runny nose, sneezing, itchy skin, rashes, and/or shortness of breath among others.

Autoimmune diseases involve a "mistake" of a different kind on the part of the immune system. In this case, immune-system cells, for reasons as yet unknown, target certain cells in the body for destruction. There are two general categories of autoimmune diseases: collagen diseases that involve the connective tissues (such as rheumatoid arthritis, which affects primarily joints, and systemic lupus erythematosus, which also may attack organs and nerve tissue) and vascular diseases (such as hemolytic anemia, in which red blood cells are destroyed by antibodies).

Where does melatonin fit in?

Since immunology—the study of the immune system—is still fairly new, it should come as no surprise that melatonin's role in this complex process is still under investigation. However, preliminary studies show that melatonin acts as an intermediary with the immune system on several different levels.

First, recent studies conducted in Locarno, Switzerland found that pinealectomy—the removal of the pineal gland and a resulting loss of melatonin—induced a state of immunodepression in rodents. When biologic amounts of melatonin were injected, however, immune-system function improved dramatically. Exactly how, and in what ways, still is unknown.

One clue lies in the fact that melatonin-binding sites—receptors on the surfaces of cells that attract and attach melatonin—have been found in the thymus and the spleen, two important immune-system organs. Furthermore, these sites are equally stimulated by adrenal hormones called corticoids, over which melatonin has been shown to have a modulating response. Some researchers believe that melatonin acts to decrease the stress-related—ultimately depleting—action of the corticoids on immune-system cells.

How else might melatonin react with the immune system?

Studies performed at the Department of Molecular Pharmacology and Biologic Chemistry at Northwestern Medical School, found that melatonin activated monocytes—large white blood cells known as leukocytes—and enhance their ability to destroy nonself cells. The same study also showed that melatonin influenced the release of IL-1 (interleukin-1), proteins that control aspects of blood-cell production and the immune response.

One animal study of particular interest showed that melatonin could restore the function of T-helper cells in mice whose immune systems had been compromised. The results of this study may someday lead to improved treatment for humans with AIDS.

(However, it should be noted that melatonin's immune-boosting capacity may exacerbate autoimmune diseases and allergies, since these conditions involve an already overstimulated immune system. This possible connection remains the subject of investigation for several researchers.)

What is AIDS?

Acquired Immune Deficiency Syndrome is caused by a virus known as HIV (Human Immunodeficiency Virus). The virus attacks a very specific subset of lymphocytes, namely the T-helper cells. Without T-helper cells to stimulate the rest of the immune system into action, the body is left vulnerable to a host of potentially life-threatening and painful infections—infections the body normally would be able to fight pretty easily if the immune system was intact. More than ten years after HIV was first isolated and the ravages of the disease first identified, scientists are searching for ways to solve what has become a worldwide crisis. To date, about 1 million Americans are believed to be infected with HIV, and another 243,000 have died since 1981; around the world, some 4 million people have confirmed cases of full-blown AIDS, another 17 million to 19 million are believed to be infected with the virus.

Apart from viruses like AIDS, what can cause an immune system to break down?

The immune system can malfunction or become depleted for a number of reasons. Certain conditions are present at birth and are a result of a genetic defect. Others are caused by nutritional deficiency and infections caused by fungi and bacteria, as well as other viruses. Certain treatments for cancer and other illnesses, such as irradiation and chemotherapy, can suppress the immune system. Severe burns and other traumas to the body, including surgery, also are known to disrupt our ability to protect ourselves from disease.

Are there substances in the environment that can affect the immune system?

As is true for virtually all other body cells, lymphocytes and leukocytes are prime targets for free-radical destruction. As Chapter Four discusses, free radicals come from a variety of environmental sources, including polluted air, electromagnetic fields, cigarette smoke, and ultraviolet rays from the sun. In fact, researchers at the University of Michigan at Ann Arbor performed a study on the effects of ultraviolet rays on the immune system. They found that skin that had been sunburned showed less reaction to allergy-causing agents than healthy skin--a sign that the immune system (which also produces allergic responses) was not functioning properly. The results of this study indicates that overexposure to ultraviolet rays can be harmful in two ways: first, by stimulating the creation of cancer cells by damaging DNA and, second, by inhibiting the immune system from recognizing and eliminating skin-cancer cells once they are produced.

Apart from taking melatonin, are there ways to boost the immune system?

Generally speaking, any habit that is good for one part of your body will help your immune system stay healthy as well.

Eat a balanced diet. Like all other body tissues, the immune system needs protein, vitamins, and minerals in order to maintain its health. Severely malnourished people are particularly vulnerable to immune-system dysfunction, so avoid processed food and go for the antioxidants in fresh fruits and vegetables.

Exercise—in moderation. Without question, regular and vigorous exercise is one of our most important life- and health-enhancing activities. And, some studies have shown a short-term immune-system boost—a rise in the number of immune-system cells—follows a bout of exercise. Other research indicates that rigorous, continuous exercise may suppress immune function over the long-term. Chances are, however, that even an ambitious exercise regimen will do far more good than harm. If you have any questions, talk to your physician.

Get seven to eight hours of sleep a night. Little conclusive research has been done on the direct effects of sleep on the immune system. However, we do know that we *feel* less well when we haven't slept, and we certainly are more vulnerable to stress.

What about stress? Does stress affect the immune system?

Absolutely, although exactly how still is unknown. In a study performed in 1990, volunteers who spent twenty minutes a day for four days writing about their worries and problems had a higher level of T cells than before the experiment began. Other studies are being conducted in laboratories all over the world to figure out exactly how our emotions are connected to our immune system.

What is psychoneuroimmunology?

Relatively new, this burgeoning and groundbreaking science studies the connection between mind and body—a connection that, although long denied by mainstream Western medicine, is quite logical. We've known for decades, for instance, that immune cells and nerve cells interact. When fighting an infection, immune cells are able to stimulate the brain to transmit impulses that produce fever. And receptors for many of the chemicals released during the fight-or-flight response, such as epinephrine and norepinephrine, have been observed on the surface of lymphocytes near the lymph nodes and in the spleen.

As examined in Chapter Ten, when we discuss how psychoneuroimmunology has been used to improve treatment strategies for cancer patients, this new science has great potential. And, Chapter Six reiterates some of the health-promoting strategies mentioned in this and previous chapters—strategies that can help you boost your natural levels of the immune-system booster, melatonin.

• 6 •

Promoting Health and Elevating Natural Melatonin

Every day, I read about something new I'm supposed to be doing to protect myself from heart disease or cancer, or to boost my immune system. Now there's melatonin. How can I keep track of it all?

It is true that health-related news seems to have become prime fodder for newspaper and television coverage of late. In some ways, of course, that's all for the best. Knowledge is power, after all, and the more you know about your body and how to keep it healthy, the better chance you'll have to live longer and, just as importantly, stay well.

Nevertheless, all this information streaming in—and a lot of it conflicting information—is apt to leave you feeling frustrated rather than inspired. One day you read that margarine is better than butter because it lowers the risk of heart disease, then a month or two later, you learn that margarine contains trans-fatty acids, which may raise levels of LDL cholesterol, the very type of cholesterol that clogs arteries.

And now you're reading about melatonin, which some researchers have proclaimed to be a "miracle" anti-aging hormone—a claim that most certainly will be dismissed by other scientists. What's the truth? The truth is, *there are no miracles*. To stay healthy and fit, and to slow down the aging process, you have to pay attention, work hard, and make a physical and emotional commitment to the process. No pill—not melatonin, not aspirin, not any new "super-cure" on the horizon—can take the place of living well every day.

That said, current studies, backed by decades of animal and laboratory research, indicate that melatonin is a crucial component of human physiology, one that popular science has largely overlooked until recently and one that we should consider when taking stock of our health profile.

Is there something special I need to do to protect my pineal gland and melatonin levels as I age?

Fortunately, the answer to that question is no—as long as you already are taking care to protect yourself from the ravages of time and the environment. That means eating right, getting plenty of exercise, sleeping well, drinking alcohol moderately (if at all), and avoiding stress when possible (and relieving it when you can't).

What about my diet? Will eating certain foods help boost melatonin levels?

Remember, until you reach the age of forty, you produce all the melatonin your body needs. Unless you suffer with a sleeping problem, there is generally no need to elevate your natural levels of melatonin. If you're over forty, on the other hand, you may well decide that taking a melatonin supplement is right for you (more about when, how much, and under what circumstances to take melatonin in Chapter Seven). The point is to make sure you have just the right amount of melatonin circulating through your bloodstream, providing all the cells of your body with its antioxidant, immune-boosting, hormone-balancing effects.

That said, the food you eat does have an impact—direct and indirect—on your production of melatonin. As you may remember from Chapter One, melatonin is derived from the essential amino acid, tryptophan. Tryptophan is found in a host of foods, including whole grains, legumes, and nuts, as well as in milk, meat, fish, poultry, and eggs. Generally speaking, then, it is fairly easy for you to get all the tryptophan you need from your diet. However, as Chapter Eight shows, eating tryptophan-rich foods about an hour before you go to bed might help to raise both your melatonin levels and the quality of your sleep.

In previous chapters, we discuss the importance of consuming antioxidant-rich fruits and vegetables while avoiding potentially toxic foods like oxidized cholesterol in connection with protecting yourself against the development of heart disease and cancer. The same general guidelines apply to preserving your pineal gland and melatonin levels. Indeed, brain cells appear to be particularly vulnerable to free-radical damage, especially as you age, so the best advice is old advice: Eat your vegetables!

I think I eat pretty well and get plenty of fresh fruit and vegetables, but I'm never sure. How can I better monitor my diet?

You're right to be concerned. A fascinating article published in *Health* magazine in October 1992 shows just how unaware most Americans are about their eating habits. Here are just a few of the ways we've been fooling ourselves:

• Seventy percent of Americans told a survey that they eat fast food less often than they did two or three years ago. But the National Restaurant Association revealed that from 1989 to 1992, the number of customers at fast food restaurants actually increased by 6 percent.

• Seventy-five percent of Americans said they eat fresh fruit more often than they did a few years ago, but the USDA reports that the amount of fruit Americans con-

sume each year has dropped by about four
pounds per person.

- Seventy-six percent of Americans claimed
they watch their diets to reduce fat, but the
USDA found that they consume almost
four pounds more fat per person than they
did ten years ago.

The best way for you to monitor your diet,
to make sure you're not fooling yourself
about the quality and quantity of food you
eat, is to keep a food diary for a week or two.
Every time you eat a morsel of food, write
down what you eat, when you eat it, and how
you feel physically and emotionally when you
decided to eat. Although this process is a bit
time-consuming, you probably will learn a
great deal about your dietary habits. If you're
disappointed by what you see when you look
back on your diary after a week or so, you
may want to talk to your physician, or visit a
nutritionist, to see how your diet might be
improved.

How do the foods I eat relate to my mood?

Emerging research sheds light on two ways
that food helps to modulate mood. First, people who experience negative emotions, such
as depression or anxiety, often seek out foods
like chocolate and other sweets to provide relief. Second, and conversely, certain foods, including sugar and caffeine, and certain eating
habits, like skipping meals or binging, may
aggravate or even trigger negative moods.
Why is there such a connection between

what we eat and our emotions? We have four main neurotransmitters in the brain that help to regulate mood—serotonin (melatonin's precursor), dopamine, norepinephrine, and acetycholine—and all of them are manufactured directly from food components. If you think about it, the old adage "you are what you eat" is perfectly accurate. In Chapter Nine, you'll find out about other ways that your eating habits may be affecting your moods, as well as how melatonin can be used to help restore neuro-hormonal imbalances that may lead to eating and mood disorders.

Will exercise increase or decrease natural melatonin levels?

That's a good question, and one that has not yet been answered definitely. One study, performed in Italy in 1992, shows that exercise does not have any effect—positive or negative—on melatonin levels, even when performed during the night, when melatonin production is at its most active.

Even if exercise has no effect on melatonin, however, you shouldn't use that as an excuse to forgo the treadmill, the tennis courts, or those Saturday morning walks through the park. The benefits of regular exercise on virtually every system of the body can not be underestimated.

I smoke cigarettes. Does that affect how much melatonin I produce?

Oddly enough, it seems that smokers actually produce a *higher* amount of melatonin than nonsmokers. In a study performed at the University of Florence, Italy, the melatonin levels of twenty smokers and twenty nonsmokers were measured at the same hour after awakening. By a small margin, the smokers out-produced the nonsmokers, at least on this one health aspect. While the causes and meaning of this phenomenon still are unknown, scientists think that smokers produce more melatonin in an effort to provide their bodies with a bit of extra protection against the nasty carcinogens and toxins they inhale with cigarette smoke. Needless to say, smoking, which contributes to the deaths of more than 350,000 Americans every year, is one of the most harmful personal and environmental habits you can have—no matter what it does to your level of melatonin production!

Can alcohol consumption interfere with melatonin secretion?

In a study conducted by the Department of Physiology at the University of Oulu, Finland, nine healthy volunteers were given ethanol (the chemical name for alcohol) to drink, each at a different time of the evening, then had their blood levels checked periodically during the night. Without question, those who drank more alcohol later in the evening secreted less melatonin—and had more trouble sleeping—than those who ingested less ethanol earlier in the evening.

As Chapter Eight discusses, alcohol may have an inhibiting effect of melatonin production, particularly if taken in excess or very late in the evening. On the other hand, moderate drinking—one or two glasses of wine with dinner, for instance—should not pose any danger to your melatonin levels or your general health over the long-term. In fact, several recent studies have shown that moderate drinking actually *decreases* the risk of heart disease, stroke, and high blood pressure, presumably by increasing HDL-cholesterol levels while helping to relieve stress. However, keep in mind that anything over two drinks a day can be dangerous. Chronic, excessive use of alcohol can seriously damage nearly every function and organ of the body.

I take medication to treat high blood pressure. Can that affect my ability to secrete melatonin?

Definitive studies still need to be completed before your question can be answered. However, it is likely that some types of anti-hypertension medication could interfere with melatonin production. Beta blockers such as proprandal, for instance, directly act upon the neuro-adrenal axis, the very system of which the pineal gland is a part.

If we look beyond the strict question about melatonin production and blood-pressure medication to consider the effects such drugs might have on sleep patterns, the answer is more clear. Anti-hypertension medication and several other common medications—prescription and over the counter—most definitely can adversely affect sleep patterns, as Chapter Eight explores.

Are electricity and power lines harmful to my health? How?

We are exposed to electromagnetic fields (EMFs)—the emissions from electricity—from the environment and from manufactured sources. The sun, and to a lesser extent, Earth's magnetic field, are the predominant sources of EMFs, but we also are inundated with emissions from radio and television communication to power lines to household appliances, particularly personal computers and microwave ovens.

The evidence that EMFs directly cause chronic diseases, especially cancer, is largely circumstantial. Because the use of electricity is the hallmark of the industrialization process, and cancer rates are astronomically higher in the industrialized world than in underdeveloped countries, scientists have considered the possibility that EMFs are involved.

Recent research has found that low-wave electromagnetic radiation (gamma waves) can split water in the body to generate the highly reactive hydroxyl free radical. By doing so, EMFs may be able to alter DNA and thus trigger the onset of certain cancers. Again, however, many scientists consider this research inconclusive.

Are melatonin levels affected by EMFs?

A study conducted by melatonin expert Dr. Russell Reiter at the Department of Cellular and Structural Biology at the University of Texas Health Center shows that nighttime exposure to light and nonvisible EMFs depressed the conversion of serotonin to melatonin within the pineal gland. Exactly why this phenomenon occurred remains unknown, but some researchers speculate that the retina—as well as being a photo-receptor sending messages to the pineal gland about light—also may be a magneto-receptor as well.

Although it's difficult to avoid electricity in this modern world, you might want to consider staying away from electric blankets at night, since EMFs from that source might directly impact your ability to produce melatonin, as well as, over the longer term, damage your body through the proliferation of free radicals.

What about X rays or other diagnostic-imaging techniques?

A recent study, performed at Jefferson Medical College in Philadelphia, indicates that diagnostic testing through X rays and other imaging techniques probably does not affect the body's ability to produce melatonin, at least if the dosages of radiation or magnetic waves remain small. In this study, eight male volunteers were exposed to three conditions between 1 a.m. and 2 a.m. on different nights: 1) a series of routine MRI (magnetic-resonance imaging studies) tests for brain imaging in dark conditions; 2) dark conditions; and 3) bright light conditions. The subjects exposed to darkness and light showed characteristic increase and suppression of melatonin secretion. As for those exposed to MRIs in the dark, they showed an increase in melatonin secretion equal to that seen in the dark control group.

Why is it important to spend some time outside every day?

Despite the ubiquitous electric light bulb, the human body still craves natural sunlight. Most artificial lighting, incandescent and fluorescent, lacks the complete balanced spectrum of sunlight and thus may interfere with the body's absorption of nutrients.

One study, conducted in 1990, shows how profound an impact lack of sunlight can have. The U.S. Navy compared the risk of melanoma—the most serious form of skin cancer—for different naval occupations. It was discovered that personnel holding indoor occupations had the highest incidence of melanoma while workers in occupations that required spending time both indoors and outdoors had the lowest rate. Although overexposure to sunlight—through tanning and burning—may be harmful, then, underexposure to sunlight appears to carry its own set of risks.

Furthermore, the sun provides the most constant and eternal signal to our body clocks, helping to create and maintain the internal balance of neurotransmitters and hormones that keeps the body healthy. When we lose this signal, we risk not only our physical, but also our emotional and psychological well-being. Such problems as low-grade and seasonal depression, sleep disorders such as insomnia and delayed sleep-phase syndrome, and even eating disorders all may be connected to a lack of exposure to natural, full-spectrum light on a regular basis.

In many of the chapters that follow, the application of light therapy to reset the body clock, relieve depression and other mood disorders, treat certain cancers, and even ease PMS are discussed. In the meantime, however, it should be stated that getting outside every day is important for your spirit and your physical being. Walking through a park or along a riverbank or even on a crowded city street connects you to nature and to the world around you in a very essential way.

What other habits are important in terms of health and longevity?

As Chapter Two outlines, a 1994 study performed at the University of California School of Public Health shows that people who followed seven simple habits—never smoking, consuming moderate or no alcohol, eating breakfast every day, never snacking, getting seven to eight hours of sleep every day, and maintaining their ideal weight—lived approximately nine years longer and suffered less disability than those who failed to practice any of them.

The good news is that simply by making one positive habit a part of your life, you'll probably end up incorporating several. According to research conducted at Harvard Medical School, for instance, women who say they drink decaffeinated coffee are more likely to exercise, buckle their seat belts, take vitamins, and eat their vegetables. Don't be afraid to start small, by making one or two changes at a time to your daily life.

One thing you may already have decided to do is explore the benefits of taking melatonin supplements. In Chapter Seven, find out about dosages, timing, quality control, and other important information about this new natural hormone supplement.

• 7 •

Using Melatonin

Who should take melatonin supplements?

Considering melatonin's potential positive effects on the body, almost every adult
over the age of twenty-five or so should at
least consider the benefits of taking a small
dose of this natural, inexpensive supplement on a regular basis. Its antioxidant and
immune system-enhancing properties may
go a long way in slowing down the aging
process, especially if you also follow some
of the healthy living tips that Chapter Six
suggests.

For people suffering from sleep disorders,
men and women over the age of fifty with
age-related sleep problems, and everybody
whose body clocks have become disrupted by
overseas travel or night-shift work, melatonin
may be the safest and least expensive remedy available.

Are there people who should *not* take melatonin?

Although melatonin supplements appear to be perfectly safe for the vast majority of men and women, it's important to understand that melatonin is a powerful hormone, and even in small doses, may affect a number of different body processes. As discussed throughout this book, the endocrine system does not work in isolation from the rest of the body or from stressors in the external environment. Although no serious side effects have been identified after decades of research, melatonin supplements are not appropriate for everyone. Talk to your doctor *before* you start taking melatonin if you are:

- trying to become pregnant,
- pregnant or breast-feeding,
- suffering from an autoimmune disease, such as rheumatoid arthritis or lupus,
- taking cortisone medication,
- coping with kidney disease.

Where can I buy melatonin supplements?

Melatonin supplements, known by the brand-name Melatone, can be purchased from health-food stores and through mail-order distributors throughout the United States. No prescription from a physician is necessary for you to purchase or use melatonin supplements.

How much do melatonin supplements cost?

Prices may vary from state to state—indeed, even from store to store—but, generally speaking, you can purchase a bottle of sixty capsules of 3 milligram supplements for about $15. Other dosages, larger and smaller, also are available for about the same comparable price. Depending on your needs, then, you could buy an entire year's supply for about $50.

What will I feel like after taking a melatonin supplement?

That depends on a number of factors: when you take it, how much you take, and your own particular body chemistry and makeup. For most people, a 3 milligram tablet or capsule will slowly but surely begin to trigger sleep-related hormonal activities within an hour or two after ingestion. Body temperature will gradually fall, production of cortisol and other stress hormones will begin to ebb, and feelings of fatigue set in. Again, these changes should be gradual and feel natural, just like getting sleepy when your body clock is working on its own. Once it's dark and you're ready for bed, the melatonin supplements boost your natural supply of the hormone, helping you to sleep more deeply than in the past.

Are melatonin supplements addictive, like sleeping pills?

Absolutely not. That's what makes natural remedies like melatonin so appealing. They work by helping the body restore and reorganize itself, allowing the body to draw on its own innate "wisdom" to put itself back into balance. Drugs, on the other hand, work by taking over the body's functions; the body doesn't work on its own but, rather, is compelled to operate by an outside source. Moreover, drugs often induce side effects—including the risk of becoming addictive—that can be avoided with the use of a natural remedy like melatonin.

After reading this book, I hope that you come to appreciate your body for its miraculous system of biochemical actions and reactions. By using natural approaches to restoring and maintaining health, you will allow your body to work as nature intended it to, and without the need for manufactured, potentially side-effect-ridden, pharmaceutical agents to solve sleep problems or other chronic conditions for which "modern" medicine often has no reliable treatment.

Has melatonin been approved by the FDA?

No, the FDA generally does not have jurisdiction over naturally occurring substances such as vitamins, minerals, enzymes, amino acids, herbs, and hormones like melatonin—as long as there are no health claims made on their behalf by their manufacturers. In other words, the laboratories that produce and sell melatonin supplements cannot proclaim that you can help prevent heart disease by taking this powerful antioxidant or even that it will help to relieve sleep problems. If they did, the FDA would consider melatonin to be a drug, subject to the same strict rules and regulations as prescription pharmaceuticals.

What responsibilities does the FDA have over medications?

The Food and Drug Administration supervises the development and marketing of all drugs sold in the United States, both prescription and over-the-counter. It is a branch of the Department of Health and Human Services, funded annually through the United States Congress, and has the authority to regulate foods, drugs, cosmetics, and medical devices that are sold between states or imported. The FDA also is responsible for ensuring that these products are pure and unadulterated, and not misrepresented through false labeling, declarations of ingredients, or net-weight statements.

There are those involved in the manufacture and sale of natural substances such as vitamins, minerals, and melatonin supplements who believe that the FDA is tied too closely to the pharmaceutical companies that create and market prescription and over-the-counter drugs. In the past, this agency has been known to assume jurisdiction over products once considered to be natural substances, but which made health claims that the FDA said could not be substantiated. In other cases, the FDA has taken natural substances off of the market that were reported to have caused harmful side effects.

I heard that L-tryptophan, an amino acid that was offered as a supplement a few years ago, caused some dangerous side effects, and was taken off the market. What happened?

L-tryptophan, a supplement made of the amino acid tryptophan (melatonin's precursor), was taken off the market in 1989 by the FDA. Until that time, millions of people had used L-tryptophan to treat depression, sleep problems, even premenstrual syndrome, safely for more than 30 years.

Then, in 1989, there was an outbreak of a rare blood disorder among some individuals taking L-tryptophan. The disorder, eosino-philia-myalgia syndrome (EMS) was linked to impurities in the supplements, as well as to immune-system weaknesses in the patients who were afflicted. About 1,500 cases of EMS related to L-tryptophan were identified, and of that number, twenty-four people died.

Eventually, the cause of the outbreak was traced to a single batch of contaminated L-tryptophan from a manufacturing plant in Japan. Nevertheless, the FDA banned all L-tryptophan supplements from being sold in the United States, a ban that remains in effect today.

What kind of screening process would melatonin have to go through if it were ever to be considered to be a drug by the FDA?

All new drugs or substances that make claims of providing health benefits undergo intensive laboratory studies, usually beginning with animal testing to make sure that the drug is safe enough to test in humans, and might provide some benefit. Once the FDA approves reports of animal tests, the drug enters into what is called Phase One, in which proper dosages, metabolism, and effectiveness is tested in ten to eighty people, usually healthy volunteers.

In Phase Two of the testing, the safety, efficacy, and possible side effects of the drug are observed in perhaps as many as 200 people, usually patients at risk of or suffering from the disease that the drug is intended to prevent or cure. Additional animal testing may be performed at this time as well.

During Phase Three of the clinical trial, researchers perform the most extensive round of tests, carefully measuring the drug's safety, efficacy, and optimum dosages in a large number of people. At this time, the drug is also compared with other drugs and with placebos to ensure that the effects seen are not due to chance or hopeful expectations. When this stage is completed, the FDA then weighs the risks and benefits of the drug before finally approving it for release.

Before the drug can go on the market, the FDA also must approve the wording of the package insert and all advertising and promotional materials. The FDA then monitors the drug's safety and effectiveness on a regular basis.

If melatonin isn't regulated, how can I be sure that it is safe?

You're right to be concerned about the quality of the supplements you take. Fortunately, the safety record for vitamin, mineral, and natural supplements—including melatonin supplements—has been consistently outstanding. According to summaries from the nation's poison-control centers, only one death (apart from the problems associated with a poisoned batch of L-tryptophan) was associated with the use of a nutritional supplement from 1983 to 1990, and that was due to overuse of niacin by a mentally unstable individual. Prescription-drug reactions or interactions, on the other hand, caused approximately 130,000 deaths *every* year during the same period.

To date, no contaminated or harmful melatonin supplements have been reported. However, as a responsible health-care consumer, it's up to you to keep yourself informed about its status through news reports and by talking with your physician or alternative health-care provider.

How long have the effects of taking melatonin supplements been studied?

Since melatonin was first isolated and identified as a hormone in 1959, virtually hundreds of laboratory studies have been performed in the United States and around the world. Research on melatonin's efficacy as an antioxidant, anti-cancer therapy, a sleep aid, a treatment for seasonal depression, and even as a birth-control agent continues to be conducted. Although none of these studies has been conducted by the FDA, they have been performed under strict scientific guidelines. To date, no serious side effects have been noted, even when the hormone is taken in very high doses.

What are some of the minor side effects that have been reported?

In general, side effects are dose- or schedule-related. In other words, some people complain that melatonin makes them feel too sleepy during the day, which may mean that the dose they're taking is too strong for their particular body chemistry. Some, rather mysteriously, find that melatonin actually keeps them awake at night, and then they feel tired the next day. The cause of such an effect could be the time they take the drug, the amount they take, or the way melatonin interacts with their individual chemical makeup. A few melatonin users report experiencing mild stomach cramps the day after taking the hormone, a phenomenon scientists think may be related to a melatonin-related increase in serotonin, a hormone closely known to stimulate smooth-muscle contractions.

How much melatonin should I take, and how often?

That depends on several factors, including your age, your body chemistry, and, most importantly, your goals. Since melatonin is a natural substance, one that will not cause serious side effects or dependency, you should feel free to experiment with dosages, timing, and frequency until you find a pattern that works well for you. In the meantime, melatonin can be taken:

- *as a treatment for sleep disorders*. If you suffer with insomnia or delayed-sleep disorder, you'll probably want to take about 3 milligrams to 6 milligrams about three to four hours before you want to go to sleep. Start with a lower dose, then work your way up if you feel it is necessary. You should take the supplements until your sleep disorder has been resolved, that is, until your body clock has been re-set and you are falling asleep at a suitable time, sleeping well until morning, and awakening fresh and ready for the day's activities.

- *as an antioxidant, immune-system booster*. If you are under the age of thirty, you should probably limit your intake of melatonin supplements to about 1 milligram a day. Even at this low dosage, it's important to time melatonin administration well. Always take the hormone in the evening, about three to four hours before you go to sleep. If you're older than 30, you may want to take more of the hormone, since your body has begun to make less and less of it naturally. Again, take it in the evening hours so that its sedative effects do not interfere with normal activity.

- *as an adjunctive therapy for cancer, AIDS, or psycho-neurological disorders*. In previous chapters, you've read about the groundbreaking studies conducted on the roles melatonin may play in the prevention and treatment of diseases like cancer, Alzheimer's disease, depression, and a host of other conditions. Chapters Nine and Ten further examine these avenues of research and how they may impact on the future of your health. You'll also find out how you and your doctor might work together to fit melatonin into your current treatment plan should you suffer from cancer or other chronic diseases.

Is it possible to take too much melatonin?

Yes in the short-term, and no in the long-term. If you take too much melatonin one night, you may well end up sleeping the next day away or at least crawling through it feeling very drowsy and fatigued. In the long-term, however, you probably won't be hurt by an "overdose" of melatonin, even on more than one night. As Chapter One cites, women involved in a clinical trial testing melatonin as a contraceptive took up to 75 milligrams every night—nearly twenty times what an ordinary person would take to help him or her sleep or protect against free-radical damage—with no side effects.

What happens if I take melatonin in the daytime?

Taking melatonin during the day may work to fast-forward your body clock, effectively making your body think it's night and time for bed. Under most circumstances, such an effect could spell disaster. When you are fatigued and sleepy, your cognitive and physical reflexes are impaired, making driving a car or operating heavy machinery risky business.

At the same time, there are several million people across the United States who can benefit greatly from a safe and effective daytime aid, namely those men and women who work the night shift. As Chapter Eight shows, it is possible for night-shift workers to avoid the feelings of lethargy and exhaustion so often a side effect of their employment.

I usually take melatonin about three hours before I go to bed. What should I do if I forget to take it on time—take it anyway?

Generally speaking, it's probably not a good idea for you to take melatonin supplements much later than usual. If you do, you'll risk setting your clock too far ahead and being unable to wake up on time, or feeling exhausted when you do. Unless you're planning to spend the next day relaxing in bed, skip one night of melatonin and get back on schedule as soon as you can.

I'm taking my teenage children on a vacation to Paris. Would it be okay to give them melatonin for a few days to help them adjust to the time difference?

Although long-term, high-dose melatonin supplementation might interfere with puberty and reproductive cycles, your teenage children—and even younger kids—might be happier, healthier travelers if they re-set their clocks quickly with help from melatonin supplements. The next chapter talks more about re-adjusting the body clock after crossing time zones.

How can I tell if melatonin supplements are working for me?

If you're taking melatonin to enhance the quality of your sleep, you should be going to bed at a time you feel is appropriate, sleeping deeply, and waking up feeling refreshed and energized. You shouldn't feel drowsy or lethargic during the day, at least not on a regular basis.

How will I know if melatonin is having any long-term positive effects, like reducing my risk of cancer and other diseases?

Unfortunately, there's no easy way to measure how well preventative, health-enhancing habits or supplements are working. Indeed, we tend to think of health only when we are ill, not when we are well. Returning the body to its natural, balanced state is the goal of using natural substances to treat disorders or as preventative tools. In fact, natural approaches are truly preventive in that they can restore function before symptoms appear. By taking melatonin to treat a slight case of insomnia, for instance, you may find that you are no longer plagued with as many headaches or infections as you once were. That's because you may have corrected more than one imbalance in the complex, interrelated neuroendocrine system.

After suffering from delayed sleep-phase syndrome for more than two years, I started taking two 3-milligram capsules of melatonin about four hours before bed about three weeks ago. So far, it hasn't really helped. I get sleepy, but not sleepy enough to fall asleep. Would it be okay to increase my dosage?

Sure. Some people with especially stubborn sleep problems have been known to take up to 20 to 40 milligrams of melatonin with no adverse effects. However, if your sleep problem doesn't resolve itself within a few weeks after you start taking a higher dosage of melatonin supplements, you should speak with your doctor about what might be at the heart of your sleep problem. In Chapter Eight, you learn about some of the medical and psychological conditions that might be having an impact on your sleep patterns and physiology.

I want to use melatonin to help protect against free-radical damage to my cells. How much should I take?

Like so many other questions asked in this chapter, this one is answered with "that depends." Since dose-related studies about melatonin's effect on free radicals have not been conducted, we aren't sure exactly how much we need to take. On the other hand, some animal studies imply that even .3 milligrams of extra melatonin may be enough to prevent free-radical damage from taking place in humans.

Again, you may want to experiment. If you're under thirty, take 1 milligram or less about four or five hours before bedtime—preferably between about 4 p.m. and 8 p.m. If it makes you sleepy before you're ready for bed, take it a bit later the next night. If you wake up feeling tired or feel sleepy during the day, you may want to cut back to .5 milligrams or less. If you're over thirty, try taking 2 to 3 milligrams a night to start and follow the same trial and error pattern until you find a dosage and schedule that fits your lifestyle and makes you feel well and rested during the day.

My doctor is very conservative, and I'm not sure she would approve of my taking melatonin to help prevent heart disease, which runs in my family. Should I tell her about it?

In general, doctors trained in Western medicine tend to look upon organs of the body as separate entities, and diseases as discreet conditions usually affecting only one or two organs at a time. Your doctor may feel more comfortable treating high blood pressure with prescription medication rather than with more natural approaches.

Ask your doctor if he or she would be willing to consider melatonin as a treatment option. On your next visit, bring this book and/or other information about melatonin so the doctor can see how much research has been done by qualified scientists. If you are unable to make headway, or for any reason feel uncomfortable with your current physician, you should feel free to choose another. Such a decision should not be made lightly, of course, especially if you've been under your current doctor's care for some time. On the other hand, only by working within an atmosphere of mutual trust and respect will prevention and treatment strategies for a chronic condition like heart disease work over the long-term.

Could melatonin interfere with any other medication I'm taking?

Melatonin is a hormone, and as such, may have widespread effects on several systems in your body. Although no drug interactions have been reported, you should discuss taking the supplements with your physician if you take other medication on a regular basis. This especially applies to corticosteroid medications, since they boost the levels of hormones that directly react with melatonin. However, please be assured that although melatonin may affect many parts of the body, its actions tend to be quite subtle and therefore, in most cases, should not interfere with most medication.

How does melatonin work with vitamin and mineral supplements?

Generally speaking, melatonin supplements will neither interfere with or enhance the actions of any vitamins and minerals you might be taking. Again, it is an organic substance that works quite naturally with these substances to create a healthy internal balance. However, as the next chapter discusses, pairing certain vitamins, including vitamins B_6 and B_{12}, as well as minerals, like zinc and selenium, may work to intensify melatonin's effect on the sleep cycle.

• 8 •

Fine-Tuning
Your Body Clock

Why are some people "morning people" and others "night owls?"

Each and every one of us has our own unique and highly individual body chemistry. Our hormonal rhythms, body-temperature cycles, and neurotransmitter activities all combine to create our personalities, regulate our physiological processes, and form our sleeping and eating habits. Some of us have internal clocks that are naturally geared to ticking later in the day, and others thrive best in the morning hours.

At the same time, it appears to be fairly easy to disrupt our natural rhythms, through either external or internal glitches in the regular patterns of our lives. Sleep disorders such as insomnia, delayed-sleep phase syndrome, narcolepsy, and sleep apnea, afflict several million adult Americans every year. Millions more work the night shift and are thus forced to live their lives in reverse. And more and more people every year take advantage of supersonic travel to cross time zones, making the world a smaller place, but wreaking havoc on their own internal body clocks.

Is it possible to reset the human body clock?

Almost always. If you need to adjust to a nighttime work schedule or travel to another time zone, for instance, a combination of melatonin supplementation and light therapy (which is described in some detail below) to advance or turn back your body clock may be quite effective. And if you suffer from a disturbing sleep disorder like insomnia or delayed sleep-phase syndrome, the same combination of treatments are quite likely to help you reorganize your sleep patterns.

At the same time, it might not be possible—or desirable—for you to try to completely change your natural body rhythms. Many people feel, and are, more productive during the morning hours than in the late afternoon; others tend to be more alert and coordinated in the evening than at any other time of the day. Unless you must fit into a particular schedule because of some urgent, external career or personal imperative, you may do better to make the most of your natural cycles by working with them instead of trying to change them. If, on the other hand, you are troubled in any way by the quality or scheduling of your sleep, you might try taking melatonin supplements and/or working with light therapy techniques to re-set your internal clock.

What is light therapy?

Light therapy is a burgeoning field of science and medicine that recognizes the importance of light—especially natural sunlight—on our body rhythms and physiology. Light therapy for circadian-rhythm disorders involves sending visible light through the eyes so that it reaches, and triggers, the pineal gland. Light stimulation, as you now understand, is the original clock-setter for most humans, helping to regulate and control a host of cyclical physiological activities.

There are several different forms of light therapy in use today; the oldest (but not always the most reliable or accessible) is sunlight itself. The sun, in fact, is the ultimate source of full-spectrum light, which means it contains all possible wavelengths of light, from infrared to ultraviolet. Generally speaking, light therapy involves the use of equipment that sheds either full spectrum or bright white light.

In most cases, the purpose of light therapy is to increase the amount of light to which we would otherwise be exposed. Why do we need more light in our lives? The fact is that the lights in our homes and our offices have a light level of only 500 lux (the international unit of illumination, one lumen per square meter), as compared to outdoor light, which has about 50,000 lux. Night-shift workers, and people who live in Arctic climates, are usually exposed to light levels of only 50 lux. Light specialists believe this "malillumination" may be at the heart of many common disorders, including fatigue, depression, skin damage, suppressed immune function, and, of course, sleep problems.

How has light therapy been used in the treatment of sleep problems or jet lag?

More and more, light therapy is being used to reset our body clocks—sometimes along with melatonin and sometimes on its own—no matter how or why they've been put off track:

- In a 1993 study conducted at the sleep laboratory of Flinders University of South Australia, bright-light stimulation in the evening delayed the phase of circadian rhythms on nine men and women who suffered from early-morning insomnia. This treatment, which involved exposure to 2,500 lux from 10 p.m. to midnight, caused an interesting reaction: Although the subjects fell asleep at their normal times, they stayed asleep an average of one and a half hours longer than usual.

- A study in Wetaskiwin, Alberta, Canada, clearly showed that students in classrooms with full-spectrum light also had less absenteeism and a higher academic-achievement record when compared with classes conducted under ordinary fluorescent lighting.

- In one study of people suffering from delayed sleep-phase syndrome, light therapy involving two hours of bright light exposure in the morning and then restriction from bright light in the evening hours, successfully altered the troubled sleepers' circadian rhythms. In addition, both sleep and morning alertness improved significantly during the treatment.

• Some people have been able to avoid, or at least allay, jet lag with light therapy. If you're planning a trip eastward—to Paris, for example—you may want to try to get up a few hours earlier than normal on the day you intend to fly. Take a walk and soak up the sun, or stay inside with all the lights on, but stay awake and surround yourself with light. Then, once you arrive at your destination, try to stay outside in the sun for an hour or two. By doing so, you may be able to move your clock forward to more closely match the rhythm of life in the new time zone.

• In an analysis of ten studies involving night-shift workers, researchers found that the circadian rhythms of the subjects could be successfully shifted after bright light exposure at night and complete darkness during the day for four days. These shifts resulted in significant improvement in both alertness and cognitive performance during work hours. In addition, the workers were able to sleep an average of two hours longer during the day.

• Other studies, which are described in Chapters Nine and Eleven, underscore the benefits of light therapy on mood disorders and other conditions, including seasonal and nonseasonal depression, eating disorders, and irregular menstrual cycles.

Do I need to buy special equipment, or visit a sleep laboratory, to derive the benefits of light therapy?

That depends on how much and for what reason you require more light in your life. For the vast majority of people, the best source of light is the one that shines down on us every day—the sun. Unless you live in a dreary or overly dark climate, you can improve the quality of your concentration, mood, and even sleep patterns by getting outside for an hour or so every day, preferably in the morning.

If your sleep or other light-related problems are more entrenched or difficult to treat, you should talk to your physician or visit a light-therapy specialist (one good source is the Environmental Health and Light Research Institute, 16057 Tampa Palms Boulevard, Tampa, Florida 33647).

Why is sleep so important?

As Chapter Three discusses, tissues in the brain and the body repair and recuperate during sleep. As an essential part of the daily human cycle, sleep is a major contributing factor in the state of your general mental and physical health. Although we can easily recover from one, two, or even three lost nights of sleep, small sleep losses, built up day after day, can result in troublesome physical and psychological symptoms. Cognitive functions decline, memory becomes impaired, reflexes falter, and moods darken and become more variable.

In fact, sleep researchers say that sleep deprivation may be the cause of many industrial accidents that seem to occur more often in the middle of the night than at any other time. The 1978 Three Mile Island nuclear-reactor accident, the Chernobyl nuclear disaster, and the Exxon *Valdez* oil spill all happened in the wee hours of the morning. And the danger from lack of sleep hits far closer to home: A 1990 study by the National Transportation Safety Board of 182 trucking accidents concluded that driver fatigue was the leading cause—ahead of drug abuse, alcohol abuse, worn tires, and bad roads.

How much sleep does the human body need to stay healthy?

That's a question medical science has not yet answered. We know how much we *like* to sleep, however. As Chapter Three cites, the majority of Americans (about 84 percent) sleep about 7.5 hours, 15 percent of Americans sleep about 5.5 to 6.5 hours, and another get about 8.5 hours of sleep. Again, how much sleep you need to maintain your health and sense of well-being remains a highly individual matter.

What is insomnia? Could a lack of melatonin be involved?

Insomnia is characterized by the inability to fall asleep or remain asleep during the course of the night. Sleep experts have identified three specific types of insomnia: sleep-onset insomnia (in which subjects are unable to fall asleep despite being tired), sleep-maintenance insomnia (in which subjects wake up in the middle of the night and are unable to fall back asleep for several hours, if at all), and early-morning insomnia (in which subjects awaken too early and feel tired during the day).

A lack of melatonin could be involved in some cases of insomnia, especially those that occur in the elderly. As you know, the pineal gland begins to shrink as we age, so that by the time we reach our fifties and sixties, we secrete very little of this essential hormone. For younger people who probably are able to secrete enough melatonin but for some reason have a disrupted circadian rhythm, melatonin supplements can be used to stimulate melatonin production at an earlier hour and provide a deeper, fuller sleep. In addition, as you'll see later in the chapter, there are several other natural remedies, involving diet, exercise, and relaxation strategies, that can help you fall and stay asleep more easily and regularly.

What is delayed sleep-phase syndrome?

If you can't fall asleep until the wee hours of the morning (from 2 to 3 a.m.), have trouble waking up, and then feel drowsy all day, you may be suffering from delayed sleep-phase syndrome (DSPS). DSPS is a form of insomnia in which sufferers prefer to sleep at hours that are incompatible with a conventional lifestyle—from 3 a.m. to noon, for instance. Although for people who are able to set their own work hours and have no other scheduled imperatives, such hours may be perfectly suitable; most of us would find such a rhythm quite disturbing.

Fortunately, treatment with a combination of melatonin and light therapy has been remarkably successful for many people wishing to advance their sleep cycles by several hours. As the study cited above suggests, bright light exposure first thing in the morning, normal activity during the day, late afternoon exercise, and melatonin supplements combined with darkness in the evening should put a DSPS sufferer on the road to recovery soon.

What else besides a shortage of melatonin could be causing my sleep problems?

Like so many other physiological activities, sleep is an extraordinarily complicated process, involving several different body systems.

Alcohol.   Although many of us think that alcohol will help us sleep, just the opposite may occur, even if you don't overdrink. Alcohol, in any amount, just before bedtime often results in a reduction of overall sleep time— including REM and non-REM sleep—and the quality of sleep throughout the night.

Medication.   The sleep process can be significantly disturbed by drug intake. Drugs that may lead to insomnia include thyroid preparations, oral contraceptives, beta blockers, and illegal substances including marijuana and cocaine, among others. In addition, a study performed at Bowling Green State University showed that aspirin and ibuprophen (both nonsteroidal anti-inflammatory medications, NSAIDs) disrupted sleep in most subjects. Scientists believe that sleep disturbance after

NSAID administration is related to suppression of melatonin and other hormone levels and changes in body temperature.

Medical problems. Gastrointestinal disorders, chronic pain, asthma, and other breathing disorders are the most common chronic medical conditions that may interfere with regular sleep patterns. That's why it's important to see your physician if you feel chronically fatigued or have difficulty sleeping for more than a few weeks.

Lack of exercise. Lethargy is defined as slugginess, torpor, and apathy. A state of lethargy often occurs in people who don't provide their bodies and spirits with regular exercise. On a physical level, the relationship between exercise and sleep involves body temperature—the higher your body temperature gets during the day, the better you'll be able to sleep at night. You'll also feel more relaxed with regular exercise, a state much more conducive to sleep than anxiety and enervation.

Food intolerance. Some people are highly sensitive to certain foods that, when ingested, cause histamine (a substance produced by the body during an allergic reaction) to be released in the brain, which may lead to sleep disturbance. Chocolate, wheat, corn, and dairy products are the most likely culprits.

How else could my diet be influencing how much I sleep?

Both eating too much (especially at dinner) and eating too little (through very low-calorie diets) can result in sleep problems. If you eat a big meal too soon before you go to bed you may be troubled by gastric problems or simply by the bodywide increased metabolism rate required for digestion.

On the other hand, low energy diets have been known to cause sleep-disturbing reductions in metabolic rate. A study, conducted at the University of Witwatersrand in South Africa, investigated the effect of a strict weight-loss diet on nocturnal body temperature and sleep patterns in young women who were overweight but not obese. After four weeks on a restricted diet, women lost 8 percent of their body weight. A majority of them showed a decline in nocturnal body temperature when measurements were taken during the last two weeks of the diet. Dieting led to a significant increase in the time before falling asleep and a decrease in the total time spent in slow wave sleep. These findings suggest that energy restriction both lowers nocturnal body temperature and alters sleep patterns.

In addition, as discussed above, food allergies have been known to cause sleep disturbances. Many sleep experts suggest keeping a food log for several days or weeks to see if you notice a correlation between a certain type of food and a problematic night of sleep.

Besides taking melatonin, how else can I work to improve my sleep patterns?

Let's review the possible causes of sleep dysfunction previously mentioned and see how you might work to eliminate them:

Alcohol.   If you are a moderate drinker, experiment a little to see if alcohol is causing your sleep problems. For a few weeks, have nothing that contains alcohol after 6 p.m. If your sleep patterns improve, it may be that you've been drinking alcohol too close to bedtime.

Medication.   If you take any medication—prescription or over-the-counter—on a regular basis, ask your doctor if there might be a relationship between it and your sleep problems.

Lack of exercise.   Make sure you're getting enough exercise—at least three times a week for 30 minutes at a time—and that you're timing your exercise correctly. Most sleep experts agree that strenuous physical activity performed about five hours or so before bedtime is most beneficial for sleep. Since this falls right after most people get out of work, you can easily add some exercise into your life by walking home, joining a nearby gym, or taking your dog (or spouse) for a brisk walk just before dinner.

However, be aware that exercise performed too close to bedtime has a counter-productive effect, since it raises heart rate and stimulates the secretion of the stress hormones, including adrenaline.

Diet.   In addition to avoiding a big meal too close to bedtime, as well as tracking possible food allergies or sensitivities, here are a few diet- and lifestyle-related tips you might want to follow:

- Certain vitamin and mineral supplements, including vitamins B_6 and B_{12} and the minerals calcium and magnesium, are known to have sedative effects on the body. Recommended dosages consist of 500 milligrams of liquid calcium, 250 milligrams of magnesium, 50 to 100 milligrams of B_6, and about 25 milligrams of B_{12}. Taken on a daily basis, separately or in combination with one another and/or with melatonin, these vitamins may help improve sleep patterns.

- Eat a small amount of protein- and/or calcium-rich food shortly before bedtime. (Tuna on two or three whole wheat crackers or a half-container of skim-milk yogurt are good choices.)

- Establish rituals, like taking a warm bath, drinking warm milk, stretching, performing deep breathing and relaxation exercises about an hour before bed, then remaining quiet until you fall asleep.

- Use your bed only for sleep, not for reading, watching television, or doing paperwork.

- Leave the bedroom to read or watch television in another room whenever you find it difficult to sleep.

- Get up at the same time every day, regardless of what time you go to bed.

- Reduce anxiety by writing down your day's problems and next day's tasks before you go to bed.

What about taking naps during the day?

The jury is divided on whether napping disrupts a good night's sleep. Some studies show that about 80 percent of people who take naps during the day don't sleep as well that night. Other people, and other cultures, swear by the health-enhancing effects of regular naps. In fact, the urge for a midday nap is built into your body clock; body temperatures and energy levels tend to fall between 1 and 4 p.m., then climb back up for a few hours. That's why we often crave sugary treats at this time of day.

If I decide to nap, when and how long is best?

If you can, take a half-hour nap during the midafternoon, say from 3 to 3:30 p.m. Naps longer than about an hour or taken much later than 4 p.m. are more likely to interfere with nighttime sleep. If you feel fatigued but are unable to fall asleep, simply lay down in a darkened room, close your eyes, and try to release any stress you feel from your body and your mind.

What about taking sleeping pills?

Every year, from 4 million to 6 million Americans receive prescriptions for sleeping pills. Although there are times when taking a sleeping pill may be beneficial—before surgery, for example, or during times of great stress or grief—sleeping pills can cause a number of side effects, including dependence, withdrawal symptoms, a hangover effect, and alteration of the memory process. Ironically, once a person stops taking sleeping pills, the insomnia that sent him or her to the pharmacy in the first place may actually worsen; this is a syndrome called rebound insomnia.

If you take sleeping pills on a regular basis, it's important that you talk to your doctor before you stop taking them. That said, you should consider finding other solutions to your sleep disorder, as well as attempting to discover the root of your sleep problems, as soon as you can.

I've been having more vivid dreams since I've been taking melatonin. Is there a connection?

Possibly. REM time is also dream time, and some people who take melatonin appear to experience longer REM sleep phases and more intense dreaming patterns than they had in the past. (For more information on the stages of sleep, please see Chapter Three.)

I work the night shift and am constantly tired and stressed-out. I also seem to get stomach-aches and headaches more often. Why is that?

More than 20 million people in North America alone work night shifts, and many of them complain of similar physical and psychological maladies. The main reason, as you already may have guessed, is that you're trying to sleep when everyone else is awake, and to work when most of the rest of your community is fast asleep.

Indeed, available information indicates that night-shift or split-shift work is associated with a number of specific health problems. Your stomachaches, for instance, may be due to disturbances of the circadian rhythm on your gastrointestinal track. Such a disturbance can disrupt the timely secretion of certain intestinal enzymes, thus resulting in excess gastric acidity. You also might want to consider your eating habits: Do you eat regular meals at regular times, or consume too much junk food on the run?

It takes the body's clock about a week to make the transition from day to night work. At first, the shift worker fights drowsiness all night long, while during the day the body, though tired, resists deep and effective sleep. If he or she is able to adapt to the new schedules and avoid giving in to miscues like morning light or other zeitgebers, they may be able to adjust within several days.

Are there other things I can do to help adjust to my new schedule?

If possible, work in bright light. Ask your employer for more light (show him or her the studies that relate bright-light therapy to increased production during night shifts). During the day, when you're at home trying to sleep, keep your bedroom completely dark and as quiet as possible. Use heavy curtains that are long enough and wide enough to keep out light. Stay in this dark, quiet environment for eight hours, whether you are asleep or not. One more trick involves maintaining the "night as day" routine even on your days off and vacation time. Unfortunately, that kind of schedule may wreak havoc on your social and family life.

What causes jet lag?

Early humans were not nocturnal and could not migrate at the speeds available today, so they did not evolve internal clocks that were up to the kind of rapid changes in rhythms and cycles demanded in today's modern world. The symptoms of jet lag—irritability, fatigue, headache, loss of appetite, irregularities of bowel movement, difficulty in concentration, among others—arise because we are attempting to match our body clock (which initially continues to run in relation to the time in the country of departure) to the new environment, with its own set of time cues (or zeitgebers).

How can I use melatonin to prevent or minimize jet lag?

At one time, sleep experts recommended that subjects take melatonin for several days before flying to another time zone. Current research, on the other hand, suggests that melatonin taken before travel can actually worsen symptoms. Instead, you should wait to take melatonin until you arrive at your destination, and then take it a few hours before you want to go to bed for the night.

What else can I do to help my body clock adjust more quickly?

To further minimize jet lag, try flying during the day instead of at night, establish a regular sleeping routine at least two days before your trip, getting at least fifteen minutes extra sleep for two nights before flying, avoid alcohol during the flight, get into the sun when you arrive, and exercise if possible. As quickly as you can, adapt to the new local hours for sleeping, being awake and active, and for taking part in social functions. Rest in a quiet dark room during local bedtime, even if you don't feel tired, and try not to nap during the day since naps may "mislead" the body into thinking it is nighttime.

I have diabetes and I'm starting to work the night shift. Are there special concerns for me?

The problems you face as a person with diabetes attempting to shift his or her body clock is more common than you think.

What's most important for you is to keep your hours—and thus your insulin injections—on a regular schedule. When you change your circadian rhythm by getting up and being active at night, you change your levels of cortisol and growth hormone. This affects your control of fasting blood-glucose levels. In addition, the stress involved with switching your circadian rhythms may well cause an increase in catecholamine levels, which could also worsen blood glucose control.

Work closely with your doctor, or with a specialist in endocrinology, to fit your medication into your new schedule. And keep in mind that the social and emotional stress you may be feeling about changing your lifestyle more than likely has had, and will continue to have, an impact on your physical self, too.

Indeed, too many of us see the mind and spirit as completely separate entities when in fact they are completely interdependent. In

Chapter Nine, you'll see how melatonin and other hormones affect your brain chemistry, and how alterations in the neuroendocrine system can affect your mood and cognitive abilities throughout your life.

• 9 •

Melatonin and the Brain

What parts of the brain work to form thoughts and create moods?

As advanced as the sciences of neurology and biochemistry have become in recent years, we still have a rather primitive understanding of the way emotions, ideas, and memories are created and stored within the human brain. Many philosophers might say that these mysterious matters are best left alone, that they are—and should remain—inaccessible to the prodding of the scalpel or the scrutiny of the microscope. Nevertheless, the search for answers to questions like this keeps neurologists and psychiatrists busy in laboratories and treatment centers around the world.

To look at the brain—a grayish-pink, jellylike ball etched with deep ridges and grooves—you probably wouldn't guess at the extraordinarily intricate activities that take place within it. Indeed, the brain is both a super computer and complex chemical factory. First, brain cells produce electrical signals that travel along pathways known as circuits; as in a computer, these circuits receive, process, store, and retrieve information. At the same time, brain function depends on the proper activity and balance of a variety of chemical substances produced by brain cells.

The brain is, in effect, the master-control center of the body. Not only is it responsible for receiving and processing information from the outside world, but it also works with other systems in the body to regulate all body activities, cognitive functions, and emotional responses.

We experience emotions through the activities of many different areas of the brain and organs of the body. A group of brain structures, called the limbic system, plays an as yet poorly understood but pivotal role in the production of emotions. Comprised of portions of the hypothalamus, thalamus, and other parts of the brain, the limbic system receives nerve impulses about emotions from other parts of the brain and body. These impulses stimulate different areas of the system, depending on the kind of sensory or thought message that arrives. The perception of anger, for instance, would involve one area of the brain and combination of responses, while joy or pleasure would stimulate and inspire others.

As for thoughts and ideas, they are processed over circuits primarily located in a part of the brain known as the association cortex. These circuits allow the brain to combine information stored in the memory with information gathered by the senses. Exactly how the brain is able to formulate abstract ideas, learn new languages, solve complex problems, and other features of higher intelligence is still a puzzle to scientists.

How do different parts of the brain communicate with one another?

Each neuron (brain cell) consists of a cell body with a number of fibers extending from it. The neuron communicates its message to other nerve cells by sending information out of its cell body through one of its hairlike fibers, an extension called the axon. All of the other fibers extending from the cell body, called dendrites, receive information from other cells.

The neuron is the functional unit of the brain. It receives information, in the form of electrical impulses, at its dendrites. The impulse first passes through its cell body, then out its axon to other neurons. The axon typically divides into a number of small fibers that end in terminals, each of which forms what is called a synapse with another cell. The synapse is actually a space between the axon terminal of one neuron and the dendrite receptor of another.

Just as a car requires oil to allow its gears to shift properly, nerve cells need certain chemicals in order for this intricate circuitry to function properly. These chemicals, called neurotransmitters, trigger the connection between the axon of one neuron and the dendrite of another.

When a neuron is first stimulated, it sets off an electrical current, which releases neurotransmitters stored near the neuron's axon terminals. These chemicals flow across the synapses to stimulate the next neuron in the nerve fiber; the process continues until the message is received by the proper center. Synaptic transmission also includes a process called uptake, in which some of the neurotransmitter molecules in the synapse are absorbed back into the nerve endings, where they either degenerate or are released at a later time.

Without the presence of neurotransmitters, neurons cannot send appropriate messages to other parts of the brain. In fact, the synaptic transmission is crucial to every body and mind action and reaction. All human activity, from orchestrating a sneeze to composing a symphony is accomplished through a series of successful synapses. The human brain, composed of more than 100 billion neurons, has at least 10 trillion synapses within it.

How many neurotransmitters are produced in the brain?

Brain cells produce as many as fifteen different chemicals that are used as neurotransmitters. Four of them—acetylcholine, dopamine, norepinephrine, and serotonin—are especially important to the regulation of brain activity.

Many researchers believe that vital aspects of our mental, emotional, and physical health are profoundly affected by the way in which these chemicals work with each other to keep the body in a state of fluid, flexible, but ultimate balance. When any part of this system becomes disturbed, physical or emotional illness may be the result.

How does melatonin fit into the chemistry lab of the brain?

As you may remember, melatonin is synthesized by the pineal gland from the neurotransmitter, serotonin. Serotonin is involved in several central physiological processes, including body temperature and blood-pressure regulation, as well as a variety of neuropsychological functions such as appetite, memory, and mood. Melatonin and serotonin are inextricably linked: When melatonin levels drop or rise for any reason, so do serotonin levels, and vice versa. As this chapter later shows, researchers are beginning to focus more and more on the role that melatonin may play in both the development and potential treatment of serotonin-related psychological and physical problems.

What are mental disorders?

Any disturbance in behavior, emotion, or cognition can be considered a form of mental disorder. According to the National Institute of Mental Health, more than 28 percent of all Americans suffer from some type of mental disorder severe enough to require psychiatric treatment at some point in their lives.

Generally speaking, there are three types of mental problems: emotional disorders, including depression and anxiety; personality disorders such as paranoia, obsessive-compulsiveness, and addictiveness; and thought disorders, which include learning difficulties, schizophrenia, and bipolar disorder. (Please note that these categories are quite flexible, and some mental disorders fit into more than one category.)

In recent decades, studies of the brain have established that many mental disorders may have a biological, chemical base much like any other organic diseases. Research suggests that the cause of some, if not most, psychological problems lies in the complex neurotransmission system of the brain, involving an imbalance among the brain chemicals.

What is depression?

Depression is the most common serious psychiatric problem in modern America, affecting millions of people each year. Depression is more than lingering unhappiness; it is prolonged and leads to a disruption of one's lifestyle and activities. Depression involves a pervasive sense of pessimism: Not only are things bad now, it seems they will be bad forever. No external circumstance, such as a visit from a friend or a vacation, will lift someone who is clinically depressed from his or her state of gloom and sadness. This "blue mood" also is accompanied by disinterest in food, work, and sex. Often, thoughts of suicide also arise. Such feelings usually are accompanied by physical changes: Sleep patterns shift, with patients either sleeping much more or much less than before, and appetite either diminishes or grows to an abnormal degree.

What causes depression?

Like other mental disorders, depression is believed to be caused primarily by a chemical imbalance of neurotransmitters. In some cases, this imbalance can be triggered by an emotional event, such as the death of a loved one or the loss of a job, and in others, depression may be a side effect of certain medication or a symptom related to another disease. No matter the underlying trigger, the end result is that brain cells are not able to communicate with one another as they should and thus the rhythm and balance we know of as mental and emotional health is disturbed.

Several different types of depression have been classified, including bipolar disorder (characterized by wide mood swings going from the depths of depression to manic euphoria), dysthymia (a mild but long-lasting depression), and Seasonal Affective Disorder (SAD), (a form of depression that occurs mostly during the winter months and may be related to a lack of exposure to natural light).

How is depression treated?

Increasingly, physicians are treating depression with a combination of psychotherapy and drug therapy. Psychotherapy helps patients explore the life situations that may have influenced the development of their disorder, while drug therapy attempts to address the chemical imbalance that apparently underlies most cases of depression.

There are several types of medications used to treat depression, and each one is designed to act on a different neurotransmitter. *Tricyclic antidepressants*, for instance, are a class of drugs that works mainly to reduce the uptake of norepinephrine—a neurotransmitter known for its stimulating effects on blood pressure, heart rate, and other body processes—and, to a lesser extent, serotonin uptake. Tricyclics tend to have a sedative effect, so much so that most patients usually are told to take their medication at night. Tricyclics are among the most frequently used antidepressants in recent decades.

Monoamine Oxidase (MAO) Inhibitors increase the action of both norepinephrine and serotonin by preventing their natural chemical breakdown. Although MAO inhibitors tend to work more quickly than tricyclics, they also involve more potentially dangerous side effects, including a life-threatening hypertensive crisis that may occur if certain foods or drinks (namely red wine and aged cheese) are consumed.

Lithium is used to treat bipolar disorder, helping to ward off the onset of mood swings. Unlike tricyclics or MAO inhibitors, lithium is not really an antidepressant but rather a mood stabilizer as effective in moderating the manic phase of the disorder as in elevating spirit during the down phase. Lithium, too, is known to have unpleasant short- and long-term side effects.

What is Prozac?

Prozac is the first of a new class of antidepressant compounds called selective serotonin re-uptake inhibitors, or SSRIs. As its class name implies, Prozac works by specifically inhibiting the uptake of serotonin at the nerve endings in the brain. This results in an increased concentration of serotonin at the synapse which, in turn, increases the availability of serotonin at the critically important brain receptor sites. Researchers and patients have been impressed by how effective this approach to adjusting neurotransmitter balance appears to be, and how few side effects SSRIs cause in most people who take them.

What is the relationship between Prozac and melatonin?

Any medication that affects the synthesis of serotonin also will affect melatonin levels. Although extensive testing of melatonin levels in patients taking Prozac have not been completed, it may well be that the benefits of a drug like Prozac, which include lifting of moods as well as improved sleeping and eating habits, also involve a boosting of natural nighttime melatonin and its incipient positive effects on the rest of the body. In fact, the benefits of Prozac may be derived not just from its direct effects on serotonin levels, but also from its indirect effects on melatonin. Indeed, if melatonin is truly the "master hormone" in charge of setting and maintaining the body's internal biological clock, then any substance that raises its level and promotes

its activities is bound to have a widespread
impact on the rest of the body.

Do people tend to be depressed more during one part of the year than another?

Seasonal Affective Disorder, or SAD, is a particular kind of depression that occurs during
the winter months. SAD's prevalence tends to
increase with geographical latitude—in Florida,
about 2 percent of the population might suffer
from it in any given year compared with 10
percent in New Hampshire. The shorter winter
days ration our sunlight, which our body clocks
need to keep our sleep/wake cycles regulated.
In addition, we know that the darker it stays,
the more melatonin than serotonin is produced
in the brain, resulting in a crucial imbalance
that may be involved in depression.

As is true for depression in general, the
cause or causes of SAD are unknown. However, we do know that when light enters the
retina, electrical impulses transmit signals to
the hypothalamus, which then sends chemical
and electrical messages about mood and emotion to other parts of the brain and elsewhere
through the body. Although melatonin levels
remain about the same among men and
women with and without SAD, most psychol-
ogists believe there may be a link between a
loss of light and the dip in mood and energy.

Could light therapy help?

As Chapter Seven discusses, light therapy
is a burgeoning new science with widespread
clinical applications for the treatment of de-

pression and other psychological and physical disorders. Full-spectrum and bright white-light therapy appears to be especially helpful in the treatment of SAD; one study shows that exposure to just one extra hour of sunlight, derived from the taking of a morning walk, dramatically lessens symptoms of SAD, perhaps by helping to restore patients' proper circadian rhythms.

Are there other psychological disorders that may be related to melatonin and/or serotonin?

Some studies have linked alterations in the melatonin/serotonin axis with schizophrenia, obsessive-compulsive disorder, and eating disorders such as bulimia and anorexia nervosa. Indeed, most common mental disturbances may involve the pineal hormone and its precursor to some degree. How could two brain chemicals be involved in so many different conditions? As discussed previously, melatonin's greatest influence on the body and mind involves its role in the body's circadian rhythm metronome. Some researchers believe that whenever this rhythm is disturbed by a lack of melatonin or, by extension, an imbalance of serotonin, a wide range of mental and physical disorders may result.

Why do scientists think that melatonin could be involved in schizophrenia or seizure disorders?

Many studies have shown that people with schizophrenia may have one or more physical brain deformities, including abnormally small pineal glands and thus limited levels of melatonin secretion. Conversely, epilepsy and other seizure disorders—the incidence of which decreases with age—may be triggered in part by overstimulation by melatonin. In fact, some researchers feel that benzodiazepines, a class of drugs often used to treat seizure disorders—may exert their anti-epileptic activity by decreasing nocturnal melatonin secretion.

What is Alzheimer's disease?

Alzheimer's disease is a degenerative brain disorder characterized by a decline in intellectual and social abilities, and particularly of memory. This disease—the cause of which remains unknown—produces abnormalities in certain areas of the brain. It is thought to account for approximately 50 to 60 percent of all cases of dementia (any disorder in which mental functions break down). The risk of developing Alzheimer's disease increases with age. It is thought to occur in approximately 4 percent of persons sixty-five to seventy-four years old, 10 percent of those seventy-five to eighty-four years, and 17 percent of those eighty-five years or older.

Is there a relationship between melatonin and Alzheimer's disease?

Recent research has shown that Alzheimer's disease patients may have abnormally low melatonin levels, raising the possibility that this disease may be related, at least in part, to the destruction of brain cells by free radicals as we age—destruction that might have been avoided had melatonin's powerful antioxidant qualities remained available to protect brain cells.

Should I give melatonin to my mother, who has Alzheimer's disease?

No definitive research studies have yet been done to prove that therapy with melatonin supplements either allays symptoms or inhibits the progression of Alzheimer's. On the other hand, we do know that melatonin is safe and has widespread beneficial effects, so there is no reason not to offer your mother melatonin. Supplemental melatonin may not only help your mother sleep better—often a challenge for Alzheimer patients—but also help reorder and reorganize her internal body clock, which often gets out of kilter with this devastating, degenerative brain disorder.

What about other degenerative neurological conditions like Parkinson's disease?

Parkinson's disease (PD) involves the loss of certain brain cells, called the substantia nigra, which are largely responsible for the production of the neurotransmitter, dopamine. Dopamine is important in the transmission of nerve impulses regulating smooth, rapid movements of the limbs and body. Without dopamine, the muscles become rigid, movements become slow and limited, and tremors are caused perhaps by an imbalance of acetylcholine, a brain chemical whose actions are usually moderated by the presence of dopamine.

The cause or causes of PD, which affects more than 1 million Americans, are unknown.

However, most scientists believe that the loss of substantia nigra cells may be due to free-radical damage, or damage by toxic substances from the environment that manage to break through the blood/brain barrier to wreak havoc on this essential group of brain cells. The steady decline of melatonin and its protective antioxidant effects as we age may help to explain the gradual nature of PD development.

Is a disease like multiple sclerosis related to melatonin?

Multiple sclerosis (MS) develops when axons in parts of the brain and spinal cord lose their myelin sheaths—their fatty, insulating covers—and are thus unable to carry nerve impulses properly. Although the cause of the disease is unknown, evidence suggests that it may have an immunologic basis. The body may make antibodies or activate lymphocytes against myelin for reasons as yet poorly understood.

Some research points to the pineal gland as the "prime mover" underlying the spontaneous exacerbations and remissions in MS. One reason this connection has been made is because the incidence of MS is highly age-dependent: It is quite rare prior to age ten, unusual prior to fifteen, and peaks in the mid-twenties. It has been suggested, therefore, that the manifestation of MS is dependent on having passed the pubertal period. Since melatonin, known to be a powerful immune-system booster, declines dramatically after puberty, its loss may somehow trigger or exacerbate the development of MS.

Can migraine headaches be treated with melatonin?

The word migraine, derived from French and Greek, means "half a head," an apt description of these headaches, which often attack one side of the head. Migraines are quite common, affecting as many as 15 to 20 percent of men and 25 to 30 percent of women. Cluster headaches, which are closely related to migraines, involve excruciating pain around the eyes and occur in periodic clusters over several days. Cluster headaches are more rare and tend to affect men more than women.

Like so many other neurological disorders, the root causes of headaches remain a mystery. More and more research, however, indicates that hormonal fluctuations and disruptions of the circadian rhythm may be involved in many types of headaches, including migraine and cluster headaches. Scientists are hoping to develop new and more effective medications, as well as preventative strategies—perhaps using melatonin supplements—based on this theory.

As endlessly fascinating and complex as the brain is, it is not the only mystery facing medical researchers. Indeed, the search to find the cause and cure for one of nature's most intransigent and deadly diseases—cancer—only intensifies with every passing year, a subject Chapter Ten takes up.

• 10 •

Cancer and Melatonin

What is cancer?

By definition, cancer is any group of cells that reproduce uncontrollably and abnormally, resulting in a growth called a malignant tumor. Abnormal cell reproduction can occur spontaneously, through some internal malfunction within the cell itself, or it can occur when the cell comes into contact with an external agent that triggers a disruption of the cell's normal activity.

As Chapter Two describes, every cell in the body normally "knows" how often and under what circumstances it is to reproduce, as well as at what rate it will be destroyed or lost in the body. This information is part of the cell's genetic code. If cells are triggered by a cancer-causing agent or otherwise malfunction, this means that their genetic code is fundamentally altered. In effect, cancer cells lack the control to stop their growth processes and therefore continue to divide without internal restraint.

At the same time, cancer cells do not die at a normal rate—in fact, they only die if they outgrow their blood supply—and thus continue to grow until they form a tumor. In addition to encroaching on the healthy tissue from which it arises, some cancer cells may travel from the original site to another part of the body. When these cells invade distant tissue, it is called metastasis. The ability of cancer cells to metastasize is what makes cancer potentially deadly.

All cancers begin with the corruption of a single cell. When that cell divides, there are two cancer cells; when they both divide, four cancer cells exist, and so on. Different cancer cells divide at various rates. The time it takes for a particular cancer to double its size is called its "doubling time." Fast-growing cancer may double in size over one to four weeks; a slow-growing cancer may take up to five years to double.

When a tumor is large enough to be seen on an X ray, it usually has to be about one half inch (1 centimeter) in diameter. At this size it will contain about a billion cells. Until a malignant tumor has disrupted the function of a vital cell or otherwise produces symptoms, the person whose cells have gone awry may have no idea that he or she is ill.

What causes cancer?

The quest to identify the cause or causes of cancer continues in laboratories and research hospitals across the country and around the world. Thanks to recent advances in medical technology and in the field of cellular biology, we are closer than ever to understanding just what happens to turn healthy cells into cancer cells, and what we can do to prevent it from happening and to reverse or slow down the process once it begins. And, as you'll see later in the chapter, melatonin plays an important role in some newly emerging cancer treatments.

In the meantime, here are a few of the most exciting theories about the pathogenesis of cancer:

• *Oncogenes*. It has often been noted that some cancers seem to "run in families." With the identification of oncogenes, scientists have been able to substantiate with medical evidence what had been merely anecdotal information. Oncogenes are genes that will act to transform a healthy cell into a cancer cell if triggered by certain agents.

Genes are chemical substances within our cells that carry blueprints for our body's structure and function. The basic component of the gene is deoxyribonucleic acid, commonly known as DNA. Approximately 10,000 pairs of DNA comprise a single gene. A number of genes together, sequenced in a certain order, make up a chromosome. It is the coded information contained in the chromosome that determines, to a large degree, how each cell develops and behaves.

New techniques in molecular biology have made it possible for scientists to see abnormalities in the chromosomes and their genes, including tiny mutations of DNA. The DNA abnormalities that lead to the development of cancer may occur in either of two types of genes—oncogenes that promote cell growth and suppressor genes that suppress cell growth. What usually stops oncogenes from being transformed into cancer-causing genes are the suppressor genes. If suppressor genes are unable to do their job properly or are missing, oncogenes may be more easily triggered to begin the process of cancer development.

• *Viruses*. It has long been suspected that viruses—tiny disease-causing organisms—may play a role in some cancers. Hundreds of times smaller than most bacteria and a thousand times smaller than the cell it infects, a virus is only able to reproduce within another living cell. After a virus enters the body, it first attaches itself to a host cell, invades it, and releases a substance that transmits hereditary characteristics from one generation to another. The virus virtually takes command of cell operations, compelling the cell to attend to its coded instructions. The instructions are to make more viruses—or to produce cancer cells.

It appears, however, that viruses do not act alone in producing cancer; not everyone exposed to a cancer-related virus develops cancer. Instead, some predisposing factors also must be involved, such as an individual's genetic background (including the presence of oncogenes or lack of suppressor genes) or environmental triggers like the ones you'll read about below.

- *Free-radical damage.* As you may remember from Chapter Four, free radicals are unstable molecules that damage healthy cells by "stealing" particles from them. This process often causes fundamental changes in the cells' genetic material. One result of these genetic alterations may be to turn a healthy cell, one that knows how often and for how long to reproduce, into a cancer cell, which grows uncontrollably.

- *Hormone imbalances.* There is much evidence to support the theory that the development of some cancers in both women and men is related to the amount of sex hormones individuals are exposed to in her or his lifetime. Many cases of breast cancer and endometrial cancer are related to how much estrogen—the primary female hormone—the organ is exposed to during a woman's lifetime. Men, too, appear to be affected by hormonal levels; prostate cancer is far less likely to develop in men who have had their testicles removed before puberty and thus do not produce the male hormone testosterone.

- *Weaknesses in the immune system.* Medical researchers are closely examining the relationship between the development of cancer and the immune system. As Chapter Five outlines, the immune system automatically goes into action to fight off any disturbance or intrusion of foreign invaders, mobilizing a defensive array of white blood cells and chemicals. Some of these elements recognize a foreign substance—viruses, bacteria, and malignant cells—as something that does not belong in the body. Other parts of the immune system then spread the alarm, trap the invader, and kill it. Researchers believe that many cancer cells are intercepted and destroyed by the immune system before they form tumors. If the immune system is somehow weakened, however, such interceptions are not made and cancer cells are allowed to live and reproduce.

- *Carcinogens*. Scientists estimate that as many as 80 to 90 percent of all cancers may be related to substances in the environment we call carcinogens. The best known carcinogen is tobacco smoke, which is linked to the most common deadly cancer in the United States today: lung cancer. Other carcinogens include radiation, industrial agents and toxic substances such as asbestos, coal tar products, benzene, cadmium, uranium, and nickel. (In a way, free radicals can also be termed carcinogens.)

- *Dietary influences*. Eating patterns may strongly affect the risk of developing cancer. Indeed, eating a healthy, nutritious diet may help reduce an individual's cancer risk by as much as 30 percent. Some things you consume promote cancer development, while others help prevent it:

    Excess consumption of alcohol may be a factor in as many as 4 percent of all cancers, particularly of the head and neck and of the liver. Alcohol is especially deadly in combination with another carcinogen like tobacco.

Some studies suggest that a *high-fat diet* increases the risk of cancer of the colon and breast, and possibly of the ovary, uterus, and prostate. One theory explaining this link proposes that a diet high in fat affects the secretion of the female sex hormones, which might influence the development of cancer in the reproductive organs. High-fat diets also increase the amount of cholesterol and bile acids that are in the colon, which may then be converted by bacteria into carcinogens.

Finally, a *low-fiber diet* has been linked to development of colorectal cancer, which is second only to lung cancer in its high mortality rate. Researchers theorize that a lack of fiber promotes colorectal cancer by slowing down the process of waste elimination through the intestinal tract.

• *Lack of exercise.* As far back as the 1920s, researchers found that desk-bound people developed more cancer than those who did physical work. Colorectal cancer—one of the most prevalent cancers in the United States today—may be especially connected to a lack of exercise, since its development may depend on the rate at which food and waste pass through the digestive system. Exercise can speed this rate up, thereby decreasing the amount of time potential carcinogens come into contact with intestines. In addition, active women produce less estrogen than inactive women, which helps to explain why those who exercise are about two times less likely to develop cancers of the reproductive system than their sedentary peers.

In the end, however, there are very few instances in which the exact cause of a specific cancer can be identified. Even lung cancer, which is directly linked to cigarette smoking in most people's minds, may be caused by another unknown factor. Not everyone who smokes develops lung cancer, nor has everyone with lung cancer smoked cigarettes in the past. Clearly, multiple factors, some perhaps not as obvious as cigarettes, must work together in order for cancer cells to be formed.

Can melatonin prevent cancer?

Research into melatonin as an anti-cancer agent is just beginning. If you have cancer, or feel you are at particular risk of developing the disease, it is important for you to learn as much as you can about other prevention and treatment strategies. Melatonin is not, and will never be, a miracle cure for cancer or any other disease.

That said, the hormone does influence many systems of the body that may be involved in suppressing the development of cancer. First, you've already read about melatonin's remarkable antioxidant properties, properties that may protect cellular DNA from

becoming damaged by free radicals and carcinogens. This protection from external damage
also might inhibit oncogene activation.

Second, melatonin also is known to be a
powerful immune system stimulator, which
may help to keep the body's defense system
alert and ready to recognize and destroy cancer cells before they have time to do any
damage.

Finally, as one of the endocrine system's
most important regulators, melatonin may
play an important role in preventing overstimulation of tissues by estrogen, testosterone, and other hormones.

How is cancer treated?

Every year, new advances are made in the
treatment of cancer—advances that have
translated into vastly improved survival rates
for most cancers. Today more than 3 million
Americans are cancer survivors—people first
diagnosed more than five years ago who are
now cancer-free. And today more than four
out of every ten new cases of cancer will be
cured (cure being defined as surviving cancer-
free for five years or more), thanks to the effectiveness of modern cancer therapy.

Surgery remains the best form of treatment,
and may even lead to an immediate cure. For
a surgical cure to be possible, the tumor has to
be localized in an organ or area of the body
that can be safely removed. Often, radiation or
chemotherapy will be administered before surgery to shrink the tumor and thus make it
more operable.

Radiation therapy is the second most common form of cancer treatment, after surgery. About half of all people with cancer need radiation treatments at some point during their therapy. Radiotherapy uses high-energy X rays, electron beams, or radioactive isotopes to kill cancer cells. Radiation is sometimes used alone to cure early-stage, localized tumors, freeing the cancer patient from the need for surgery. More often, it is used to reduce the size of a cancer before surgery or to destroy any remaining cancer cells after surgery.

Chemotherapy kills cancer cells through the use of drugs or hormones. Taken either orally or through injection, chemotherapeutic agents are used to treat a wide variety of cancers. They may be given alone or in combination with surgery, radiation, or both. Chemotherapy destroys hard-to-detect cancer cells that have spread and are circulating through the body. In fact, of the three basic cancer treatments, chemotherapy is the only one able to treat cancer's most lethal weapon—the ability to metastasize or spread through the body. Chemotherapy has the advantage of traveling in the bloodstream to almost all parts of the body, and thus is able to eradicate cancer cells that are out of reach of the scalpel or radiation beam.

What new ways are being developed to treat cancer?

Every day, cancer researchers come closer to finding a cure to this disease. Although the ultimate goal has not yet been achieved, enormous progress has been made in finding more effective treatments that have fewer side effects than standard therapies. Among the new avenues in cancer treatment perhaps the most promising is biological therapy, which attempts to use the body's own immune system to track down and eliminate cancer cells.

Until recently, it appeared that the immune system could not recognize cancer cells as foreign, perhaps because there are so few differences between normal and tumor cells. Biological therapy attempts to strengthen the immune system and improve its ability to destroy cancer cells. It is in this avenue of cancer-therapy research that melatonin plays a large role.

Although some forms of biological therapy remain under investigation, others have become accepted treatment for some cancers. The therapy consists mainly of treating the immune system with highly purified proteins—complex compounds made up of amino acids—that help activate the system or help it do its job more effectively. Two of the most promising forms of biologic therapy are the following:

1. Interferons and interleukins are cytokines—molecules that normally work to facilitate communication between immune-system cells. Research has found that with injections of interferons and/ or interleukins the immune system becomes more active and thus may work to destroy tumor cells. Interferon has been shown to be effective against some forms of kidney cancer, melanoma, and

leukemia. The effects of interleukin therapy are less well known, but some kidney tumors and melanomas have responded to injections of this immune-system stimulator.

2. Colony-stimulating factors do not work directly against tumors, but instead trigger the action of certain immune-system cells—called macrophages, monocytes, and neutrophils—that usually provide the body's first line of defense against foreign substances. If the amount of these cells can be boosted, researchers feel the patient's body will be able to tolerate higher dosages of chemotherapy and radiation without succumbing to serious infections caused by the loss of white blood cells.

What role might a combination of interleukin-2 and melatonin play in cancer therapy?

For reasons not yet well understood, melatonin and interleukin-2 (IL-2)—a natural protein involved in the immune response—may combine to form a powerful anti-cancer agent. Studies have shown that melatonin may either enhance the immune effects of interleukin-2 itself, or make the cancer cells themselves more susceptible to the actions of interleukin-2. Results of studies performed in Milan, Italy, show that the immune system-boosting action of melatonin may in fact involve the stimulation of T-helper cells, which then trigger interleukin-2 to produce macrophages and other immune-system cells.

These same scientists, working at the Division of Radiation Oncology at San Gerardo Hospital in Milan, found that a combination therapy consisting of low-dose IL-2 and melatonin offered some hope to patients with advanced, hard-to-treat solid tumors. A high percentage—more than 30 percent—experienced either some real improvement in the course of their disease or at least did not progress as fast as they might have without the treatment.

What is estrogen-receptor-positive breast cancer?

Breast cancer remains one of the most common and potentially deadly cancers among women, second only to lung cancer. Recent research has identified two very different types of breast cancer—cancer cells that appear to be *stimulated* by the presence of estrogen, and cancer cells that appear to be *unaffected* by the presence (or absence) of estrogen.

Can melatonin play a role in the treatment of estrogen-positive breast cancer?

In a study performed at the Tulane University School of Medicine in New Orleans, scientists grew human breast-cancer cells in the lab and then added melatonin to some of the cultures. They found that estrogen-receptor cells treated with melatonin grew one-quarter to one-half as fast as untreated cells did. The fewer estrogen receptors a batch of cells had, the more melatonin it took to retard their growth, and the hormone had no effect at all on cancer cells that lacked estrogen receptors.

What is the relationship between melatonin and the drug tamoxifen?

Tamoxifen is an established recurrence-blocking drug that is being tested nationally as a means for preventing the initial development of breast tumors. Additional studies have found that melatonin boosts the ability of the drug tamoxifen to inhibit the growth of human cancer cells in the laboratory. Melatonin might eventually be used with tamoxifen or combined with chemotherapy agents so that lower-dose, less toxic chemotherapy can be used.

Is melatonin effective in treating another type of estrogen-dependent cancer?

Like estrogen-dependent breast cancer, certain cases of endometrial cancer—cancer of the lining of the uterus—may be caused or exacerbated by prolonged exposure to estrogen. Too much estrogen can cause a buildup of endometrial cells, a condition known as hyperplasia. Hyperplasia can develop into endometrial cancer if the cells are not sloughed off every month during regular monthly menstruation. Such a buildup can occur if estrogen levels are abnormally high or levels of progesterone—the other main female hormone responsible for triggering the shedding of the endometrium during menstruation—are low.

Although research continues to discover if melatonin may play a role in decreasing the risk or slowing down the development of endometrial cancer, researchers remain hopeful. Melatonin not only has anti-estrogen properties, but also appears to stimulate progesterone, the other main female hormone that works in opposition to estrogen.

How long before melatonin could become part of standard protocol?

As Chapter Seven discusses, the process by which a new drug or drug treatment must pass through before being available to the general public often is a long and complicated one. These clinical trials are conducted under stringent conditions after years of laboratory research and, often, animal testing. So far, no standard treatment protocol involving melatonin has reached Phase One of clinical trials.

What other types of cancer has melatonin been used to treat?

Scientists are investigating the use of melatonin in the treatment of inoperable brain cancers. A study reported in the February 1, 1994, edition of *Cancer* shows that patients given melatonin (20 milligrams a day at 8 p.m. orally) along with supportive care (steroids and anti-convulsant agents) were found to survive longer and to be free from cancer progression longer than patients treated with supportive care alone. In addition, complications were significantly more frequent in patients treated with supportive care alone than in those concomitantly treated with melatonin. Therefore, it seems that melatonin may be able to improve both the survival time and the quality of life in patients with brain metastases due to solid tumors.

Furthermore, research conducted in Italy and the United States has found that melatonin also has improved survival rates and quality of life in patients suffering with hard-to-treat colorectal and lung cancers.

I've recently been diagnosed with advanced liver cancer. I asked my doctor about treating me with melatonin along with chemotherapy, but he knows nothing about it. What can I tell him?

A study published in the February 1994 issue of *Cancer*, the journal of the American Cancer Society, may be of interest to you and your doctor. It shows that both the progression of most cancers, including liver cancer, and the side effects of chemo- and biologic therapy, were severely diminished in patients who were given melatonin. The results of this study, and the others mentioned in this chapter, point to the enormous potential of melatonin in cancer treatment.

Again, however, it must be stressed that research into melatonin as a treatment for cancer is just beginning. Indeed, the conclusion of the article in *Cancer* states that, although the results are encouraging, much more research needs to be done before melatonin can be considered part of any standard medical treatment for cancer.

What role could emotions play in cancer prevention or treatment?

"The best inspirer of hope is the best physician," wrote the nineteenth-century French neurologist, Jean-Martin Charcot, a doctor as much renowned for his powers of observation as his medical techniques. Today, after several centuries of shunting aside the power of hope in favor of medical technology, more and more modern physicians are realizing how important the human spirit is to health and to the battle against disease.

Several studies have shown not only that the mind/body connection exists, but that it may be a very powerful force in fighting disease. In 1989, the results of a study confirmed what many physicians and patients had believed for some time—that the emotional support provided by cancer-support groups affected in a positive way the outcome of treatment. Dr. David Spiegel, a psychiatrist at Stanford University, divided a group of eighty-six women, all of whom had metastatic breast cancer. One group was given standard medical care—surgery, chemotherapy, and radiation. The members of the other group received the same therapy but also were asked to meet once a week in a group-therapy session in which emotions—often dismissed by physicians concentrating on the strictly physical aspects of cancer—were expressed, discussed, and confronted.

The immediate effects surprised few people: the women who had the support of fellow cancer patients and a qualified leader reported fewer symptoms of depression, anxiety, and pain than those in the other group. After all, they had more opportunities to express their emotions and find solutions to problems.

What did surprise Spiegel and other physicians were the long-range effects of support groups. Several years later, Spiegel made a startling discovery: Those who took part in the group psychotherapy lived twice as long after they entered the study as the group that received only standard medical care.

Another study, conducted in the 1980s at the Malignant Melanoma Clinic in San Francisco by psychologist Lydia Temoshob, shows similar results. Cancer patients who displayed an overreaching need to be in control and who were unable to express their emotions (whom Temoshob termed Type C patients) did not respond as well to treatment as did their more expressive and more relaxed counterparts.

One of the most famous and well-documented studies of the mind/body connection and cancer patients was performed in the late 1970s by Dr. O. Carl Simonton and his wife, Stephanie Matthews-Simonton. The Simontons developed a meditation and visualization program to help men and women with cancer tap into the power of their own emotions. In an interview for the book, *The Practical Encyclopedia of Natural Healing*, Dr. Simonton states his beliefs this way, "You [the cancer patient] may actually, through a power within you, be able to decide whether you will live or die, and if you choose to live, you can be instrumental in choosing the *quality* of life you want." In 1979, the Simontons published a study that shows that people with cancer who allowed their minds and emotions to play a role in the treatment of cancer lived *two times* longer than those who received medical treatment alone.

Cancer remains one of the nation's most intransigent health concerns, but one for which new advances are being made every day. By focusing on the profound role of hormones, like estrogen and testosterone—and, yes, melatonin—scientists have opened the door on a new world of cancer research. Chapter Eleven examines the role melatonin may play in another important health arena: women's reproductive health.

• 11 •

Melatonin
and the Female Cycle

What impact does the endocrine system have on a woman's overall health?

Hormones play a critical role in determining the quality—and perhaps even the longevity—of a woman's life from the time of her birth through her productive years and beyond. To a large extent, hormones determine whether a woman will be fat or thin, tall or short, calm or nervous, fast-moving or slow, healthy or plagued by major and minor illnesses.

What hormones are involved in the process of reproduction? And does melatonin play a role?

The endocrine glands primarily responsible for sexual development and procreation are called the gonads. In men, the gonads are called testes or testicles, and these glands produce the male sex hormone testosterone. In women, the gonads are ovaries, two glands comprised of smooth muscle located in the lower abdomen, one on each side of the uterus. The ovaries produce and store eggs, as well as secrete the female sex hormones, estrogen and progesterone. In addition to the primary gonads, estrogen also is produced by the adrenal glands, which are located on top of each kidney.

Melatonin receptors have been found on cells within the ovaries, as well as on the adrenal glands themselves. Although the exact role that melatonin plays in the reproductive system is still uncertain, researchers believe that levels of the hormone in the bloodstream trigger major lifecycle events, like the start of puberty and the end of menses, as well as help regulate and moderate the effects of estrogen on the body.

What happens to hormone levels during a typical menstrual cycle?

A female child is born with ovaries that are completely stocked with all the eggs she will ever have—about 1 million. During her fertile life, a woman will release just 300 to 400 eggs—one each month for thirty-five to forty years. The rest simply atrophy. At the time a woman enters menopause, only about 10,000 eggs remain.

Every month, a woman's body prepares one egg (or sometimes two) for fertilization and the uterus for a potential pregnancy. This preparation is called the menstrual cycle, and it is largely orchestrated by the secretion of certain hormones. The average cycle lasts twenty-eight days, roughly divided into the estrogen phase and the luteal phase.

The Estrogen Phase.   At the beginning of the cycle, the hypothalamus sends a message in the form of a hormone called gonadotropin-releasing hormone (GnRH) to the pituitary gland. The pituitary, which is located just below the hypothalamus, then relays its own message to the ovaries through yet another chemical messenger called follicle-stimulating hormone (FSH).

Stimulation from FSH causes one of the follicles in one of the ovaries to grow and the ovum within it to mature. At the same time, a thick layer of cells covering the follicles secretes a type of estrogen called estradiol. Released into the bloodstream, estradiol acts on the lining of the uterus (the endometrium), causing it to grow and thicken in preparation for the arrival of a fertilized egg. This occurs during the first part of the cycle, called the estrogen phase, which lasts about fourteen days.

The Luteal Phase.   On or about the fourteenth day of the cycle, the hypothalamus, stimulated by elevated estrogen levels, signals the pituitary to secrete a second hormone, known as luteinizing hormone (LH). The surge of LH causes the developing follicle to enlarge and rupture. In an event known as ovulation, the mature ovum is then expelled into the Fallopian tube and makes its way up into the uterus, a journey that takes about six days. While it is in transit, the egg can be fertilized if sperm are present.

In the meantime, the remnant follicle in the ovary is transformed into a working endocrine gland called the corpus luteum. The corpus luteum produces both estrogen and large quantities of progesterone, the sex hormone dominant in the second half of the cycle. Under the impact of progesterone, the cells in the uterine lining grow and mature. By the end of the menstrual cycle, the endometrium has doubled in thickness, and large amounts of nutrients meant to nourish a fetus have been stored there.

In most cases, the egg is not fertilized and hormone secretion within the uterus ebbs. The corpus luteum begins to shrink and levels of estrogen and progesterone drop. When the hormonal level is at its lowest, the uterus sheds its lining and what is known as the menstrual period begins. By the fourth or fifth day, hormone levels have dropped enough to signal the hypothalamus to resume the process.

What happens if an egg is fertilized?

If sperm is present and the egg is fertilized, the fertilized egg implants itself into the lining of the uterus called the endometrium and a special hormone, called chorionic gonadotropin, is secreted to stimulate the continued production of estrogen and progesterone.

What is PMS?

The hormonal changes during the menstrual cycle prompt a number of subtle physical changes affecting almost every organ and system in the body. For some women, these changes cause uncomfortable side effects. During the estrogen phase, for instance, high levels of estrogen increase salt and water retention causing breasts, fingers, feet, and the abdomen to bloat. During the luteal phase, when progesterone levels are high and the endometrium begins to thicken, there may be cramping. Constipation or, alternately, diarrhea also may occur during the premenstrual period, as may headaches (especially migraines), food cravings, and mood swings.

How can PMS be treated, and is there a role for melatonin?

Generally speaking, physicians don't recommend that women attempt to adjust their hormone levels by taking medication. Ibuprofen or other nonsteroidal anti-inflammatory drugs are quite effective in preventing or relieving menstrual cramps for up to 90 percent of all women who suffer from them. These drugs block the production or action of prostaglandins, hormonelike substances that are produced in many body tissues and which seem to have numerous functions—including a role in producing uterine contractions. Researchers have found that menstrual blood contains high levels of prostaglandin, which may cause excessive contraction of uterine muscles, squeezing shut the blood vessels that bring oxygen to the muscle and thus resulting in pain.

Interestingly enough, melatonin, too, is

known to have an inhibitory effect on the production and behavior of prostaglandins. Whether or not taking melatonin supplements during the menstrual cycle will work to prevent or alleviate PMS, this action could translate into a reliable and effective treatment.

How do birth-control pills work?

Generally speaking, oral contraceptives contain compounds related (but not identical) to estrogen and progesterone. If taken orally, these hormones go from the digestive tract into the liver, which breaks them down. Synthetic hormones used in oral contraceptives, on the other hand, travel intact through the liver into the main circulatory system, where they effectively shut down the reproductive cycle. Because of these hormones in the blood, the hypothalamus is not stimulated to trigger the production of FSH and LH. Ovulation ceases and, thus, pregnancy cannot occur. Even if ovulation does occur, implantation of the ovum is impossible because the uterus is unprepared.

Are birth-control pills dangerous?

For most women, the oral contraceptives available today do not pose very high health risks and, in fact, offer some real benefits. In the past, however, that wasn't the case. Until about ten years ago, birth-control pills contained high dosages of estrogen which, as Chapter Ten explains, may promote certain cancers, particularly of the breast and endometrium. Today, however, oral contraceptives contain progesterone as well, which offers protection against these and other types of reproductive cancers.

However, that said, current oral-contraceptive compounds are not for everyone. Women who smoke, have high cholesterol or high blood pressure, or who have had cancer of the reproductive system or the breast probably should not take birth-control pills.

Could melatonin be used as a contraceptive?

It has been observed that melatonin may slow down the pituitary gland's initial secretion of GnRH, the hormone that first triggers the menstrual cycle into motion. Researchers are working to develop a birth-control pill that uses melatonin's moderating influence on GnRH.

Scientists who study the breeding patterns in the animal kingdom have noted that GnRH may be active or inactive during different seasons of the year, apparently depending on the amount of light that enters the retina-pineal nervous pathway and causes the release of melatonin from the pineal gland at night. The duration of the nighttime release of melatonin is longer in winter than in summer; the prolongation of night, therefore, may well act as the endocrine signal to cease GnRH production. When it is springtime, and mating season, the endocrine signal for GnRH production is again "switched on" by longer hours of sunlight.

Assuming that humans are not seasonal breeders due to some kind of impairment along the retina-pineal gland pathway, researchers are looking for a way to use melatonin's obviously profound effects on the reproductive system to develop a safe contraceptive, one based on a more natural circadian-rhythm moderation.

Is such a pill available in the United States today?

The birth-control potential of melatonin is being tested in a large Dutch trial that began in about 1992. So far, more than 1,200 women have taken the combination melatonin/progestin pill. There have been no serious side effects, and the pregnancy rate has been as low as that for current oral contraceptives.

Because the melatonin pill contains no estrogen, it may be a safe alternative for women advised not to take estrogen/progestin pills because they're over thirty-five or have a history of cardiovascular disease, clotting problems, or certain cancers. Unfortunately, it may be several years, if not a decade or more, before a melatonin-based contraceptive is available in the United States.

I'm in my late thirties and my husband and I are trying to get pregnant. Is it safe for me to be taking melatonin if I'm trying to conceive?

Although taking a small dose of melatonin to help you sleep probably wouldn't adversely affect you, there is a slight chance that it could upset your cycle just when timing is most important. As you know, the older you are when you attempt to get pregnant, the more difficult it may be. Therefore, why add even the smallest risk of a disturbance to your exciting venture?

I am forty-one years old and pregnant. Should I be taking melatonin? Is it safe for my baby?

Although it's doubtful that a small amount of this natural substance would have any harmful effects on your baby, sufficient research on this aspect of melatonin supplementation has not been done. Talk to your obstetrician and personal physician for advice before taking any supplement—even vitamins.

What is menopause?

The word menopause comes from the Greek *mens* (monthly) and *pause* (to stop). Although the word menopause actually refers specifically to the very last menstrual period a woman experiences, we tend to use it to describe the whole range of symptoms that precede and follow the end of a woman's fertile life.

The average woman of the late twentieth century is fertile for about forty years, roughly from the age of twelve to about fifty-two. As early as her mid-thirties, however, her hormonal cycle may begin to change and her fertility to diminish. Not only is her store of eggs depleted, but the follicles that remain are less sensitive to hormonal stimulation from FSH and LH.

If an egg is not released during ovulation, progesterone, which depends on the empty follicle for production is no longer secreted.

Although estrogen levels also drop, the ovaries, adrenal glands, and fat cells still are able to produce some estrogen. The uterine lining, then, is being stimulated exclusively by estrogen. It continues to grow until it lacks a blood supply, which can take several months. This can result in one or more missed periods, followed by a heavier than usual cycle. Eventually, periods stop altogether and menopause is achieved.

In addition to ending a woman's fertile life, the drop-off of hormonal production associated with menopause can result in a number of often unpleasant symptoms and side effects. Hot flashes are the most common side effect of menopause, affecting about 75 percent of all menopausal women. Hot flashes occur when the hypothalamus, frustrated by its attempts to stimulate ovarian function, becomes overstimulated, resulting in the secretion of the powerful neurotransmitter norepinephrine, which causes the heart rate and body temperature to rapidly rise.

What about using melatonin as part of hormone replacement therapy for post-menopausal women?

Because estrogen increases a woman's risk of endometrial cancer, doctors recommend that women who have not had a hysterectomy use estrogen and progestin because progestin induces the uterine lining to slough off, preventing cell accumulation and cancer. Unfortunately, some studies show that adding progestin to the regimen diminishes estrogen's protective effect against stroke and heart disease. In studies now underway, scientists are attempting to find out whether or not pairing melatonin with estrogen would yield a low-dose estrogen therapy that could ease menopausal symptoms and protect against cardiovascular disease without raising a woman's risk of uterine cancer.

Is there any relationship between melatonin and osteoporosis? Could taking melatonin help prevent this disease?

Osteoporosis, a bone-thinning disease largely affecting post-menopausal women, may result in part from the body's inability to properly synthesize calcium and magnesium—a process believed to be regulated by the presence of melatonin and that appears to slow as the amount of melatonin decreases with age.

Whether or not melatonin supplements could help prevent or reverse osteoporosis is a matter still under investigation. However, combined with light therapy to help provide the body with adequate levels of vitamin D, melatonin supplements could certainly help bolster a woman's ability to synthesize calcium, magnesium, and other minerals necessary to repair and maintain strong bones.

As I've gotten older, I tend to gain weight during the winter—and a lot more than my husband does. Why might that be?

Just like many animals in nature, women apparently also have a seasonal tendency to gain weight. A recent study of 125 post-menopausal women showed significant increases in bone and muscle mass after the summer-fall period and significant decreases after the winter-spring period, while fat tissue decreased during the summer and fall and increased through the winter and spring. These seasonal differences were observed in the women's arms, legs, and trunks, and were unrelated to levels of physical activity.

Scientists theorize that the body's varying composition may be influenced by seasonal changes in the activity of the brain's hypothalamus-pituitary area—the very area most affected by melatonin. As we've discussed, this area regulates several major body hormones, such as the sex, growth, adrenal, and thyroid hormones. By the end of the year, the women had a net loss of muscle in their legs and a net gain of fat in their trunks.

As Chapter Three discusses, however, seasonal and circadian rhythms are just as vital to the health of men as they are to women. In fact, many scientists believe that the next revolution in health science will involve chronobiology, the mapping and utilization of our natural patterns of life. In Chapter Twelve, we look at some of the advances being made in this emerging area.

• 12 •

The Future of Melatonin

Will aging ever become a thing of the past?

Probably not. As far as we know, every living thing in the universe has a life cycle that includes aging and then, finally, death. And the truth is, we probably wouldn't want to eliminate this natural pattern altogether since it is, at least for now, the only way we know how to keep the environment in a relative state of balance and to make room for future generations. On the other hand, great strides have been made, and continue to be made, in extending both the number of years of human life, and the quality of the life that is lived.

Is it possible that medical science will ever develop cures for cancer, heart disease, and other major health problems the way it did for so many infectious diseases?

Again, probably not. Diseases like cancer are very complicated, involving many different combinations of physical, environmental, and lifestyle factors. An infectious disease, such as small pox, is quite specific and easy to target: once you develop and administer a vaccine against it, the population is safe. A disease like cancer, however, has no one single cause, treatment, or possible cure.

What avenues of current research look most promising in terms of offering us longer, healthier lives?

We've talked about some of them throughout this book. One of them is the work that is being done in the area of antioxidant strategies and preventative therapies against free-radical damage to body cells. Another important field that continues to emerge and that may lead us to healthy and more balanced lives is the science of psychoneuroimmunology—the science that explores the very real and quite profound connection between mind and body through brain cells, immune-system cells, our emotions, and the chemicals that allow them all to communicate. The science of genetics—particularly genetic engineering—also is filled with possible avenues for anti-aging researchers to explore.

Are there any "new diseases" like AIDS that melatonin may affect?

We know already that the immune-system deficiency involved in AIDS may be alleviated with melatonin in some patients. However, so far, the role for melatonin in the treatment of other types of infectious diseases remains relatively unexplored. It is only in recent years, after all, that melatonin's widespread influence on the body became known to scientists and physicians. Now comes the hard part: applying what we know about melatonin in the laboratory and within limited and controlled populations to the unpredictable "real" world of human disease. No doubt the experience we have with the treatment and eventual prevention of AIDS will tell us a great deal about the immune system in general, and melatonin's potential role in particular.

I've been hearing a lot about other anti-aging hormones, like DHEA. Is it related to melatonin?

As previous chapters discuss, some of the most exciting research emerging from medical laboratories around the world involves the study of the endocrine system and its pervasive influence on our health in general, and on the process of aging in particular.

Recently, a hormone known as DHEA, or dehydroepiandrosterone, has garnered attention as a potential anti-aging solution that may act much like melatonin on the body. DHEA is produced by the adrenal gland, which secretes many other hormones, including epinephrine and norepinephrine. Men and women have similar blood levels of these substances, which play a role in the formation of sex hormones such as testosterone and estrogen.

Like that of melatonin, DHEA production

rises and falls as we age. It is high during fetal development, rises during adolescence, reaches maximum levels at about age twenty-five, and declines after that. Its loss, some scientists postulate, may promote some of the changes associated with aging. DHEA has been found to boost the immune systems of patients given the substance by injection, as well as inhibit free-radical damage to brain cells, skin, and other tissues. However, unlike melatonin, the DHEA available to consumers in health-food stores does not appear to be of sufficient strength to provide these benefits and thus, for now at least, does not offer the same protection against aging as do melatonin supplements.

What is the best way for me to protect myself against premature aging?

The best advice is to live well every day. This may sound like a weak cliché, but the fact remains that every second lived is precious, every morsel of food eaten a gift, every movement your body makes a miracle, every idea and emotion you feel and express a wonder. By appreciating your body—and by providing it with all the ingredients it needs to function in harmony—you will do more to increase your longevity than taking any pill ever could.

And what are these ingredients. This book has discussed them all, but they're worth repeating:

- *Good food*. Not only does that mean ingesting a high-fiber, low-fat diet, but it also means taking the time and giving yourself the emotional space to enjoy the sensual pleasure of eating, of sharing meals with loved ones, of really tasting your food instead of fretting too much about its nutritional value (or lack of it).

- *Plenty of rest*. And that involves more than just getting your nightly eight hours of sleep. Rest also is relaxation, which means taking time to let your body and mind unwind—not only on weekends or for two weeks of vacation out of fifty-two weeks in the year. Every day without fail, reach for that place inside you that is quiet, that is connected to the rhythm of nature, and your life is bound to have more meaning as well as more vitality.

- *Hope and positive energy*. "You are what you eat" is one adage that has proven to be true. Another one that may hold some resonance in the near future is "You feel what you think you feel." Indeed, as mentioned just a few pages ago, what you perceive about your health and your body, and the way you look at the world and your place in it, may have as much to do with how successfully you pass through middle age into old age, and finally to the end of your life as anything else.

In the end, then, at least for now, it may be best to consider not just quick-fix remedies to increase your lifespan, but also to focus on those habits and substances that can improve the quality of the life you lead every day. By following healthy habits, like those mentioned here and throughout the book, as well as taking melatonin supplements and other helpful aids, you can take an active, positive role in extending your life and enriching its value.

Glossary

(Words in italics are defined within the Glossary)

Adjuvant chemotherapy. Chemotherapy used along with surgery or radiation therapy. It usually is given after all visible and known cancer has been removed by surgery or radiotherapy, but is sometimes given before surgery. Adjuvant chemotherapy usually is used in cases where there is a high risk of hidden cancer cells remaining and may increase the likelihood of cure by destroying a small amount of undetectable cancer.

Aerobic exercise. Physical exercise that relies on the intake of oxygen for energy production.

AIDS (Acquired Immune Deficiency Syndrome). A set of infections that beset a person whose immune system has been damaged by a virus known as HIV (Human Immunodeficiency Virus).

Alzheimer's disease. A brain disease associated with diffuse degeneration of brain cells, occurring mostly in middle or old age. Its cause is as yet unknown.

Amino acids. Building blocks of protein molecules that are necessary for every bodily function. Essential amino acids are not produced in the body but are essential for growth and development. Nonessential amino acids are those that the body synthesizes itself.

Antibody. A protein produced in the body in response to contact with an *antigen*. It has the specific capacity of neutralizing (creating *immunity*) to that antigen.

Antigen. Any substance recognized as "foreign" or "nonself" by the immune system.

Antioxidant. Chemical molecules that prevent oxygen from reacting with other compounds to create *free radicals*. They protect cells from being damaged.

Arteries. Blood vessels that carry oxygenated blood away from the heart to nourish cells throughout the body.

Aspirin (acetylsalicylic acid). A drug that reduces inflammation and fever. Also known to affect the platelets in the blood to prevent thickening or clotting.

Atherosclerosis. A disease of the arteries in

which fatty plaques develop on the inner walls, thus narrowing the passageway.

B cells. White blood cells that produce *antibodies* to create *immunity* against certain diseases.

Bone marrow. The soft, fatty tissue that fills the cavities of the long bones of the arms and legs; certain immune-system cells are formed within bone marrow.

Cancer. A group of diseases characterized by the uncontrolled growth of abnormal cells, which can occur in any organ or tissue of the body—and may spread to other parts of the body as well.

Carbohydrates. The sugars and starches in food. Carbohydrates are the main source of energy for all body functions and are needed to process other nutrients. Complex carbohydrates are composed of large numbers of sugar molecules joined together, and are found in grains, legumes, and starchy vegetables.

Carcinogen. Any substance capable of causing *cancer*. Environmental carcinogens include chemical agents (i.e., arsenic, coal tar), physical agents (radiation, ultraviolet rays, asbestos), as well as hormones and viruses.

Cardiovascular system. The heart together with the two networks of vessels, arteries and veins. Transports nutrients and oxygen to the tissues and removes waste products.

Catecholamine. A group of chemicals that work as *neurotransmitters*. The main catecholamines are dopamine, epinephrine, and *norepinephrine*. They are responsible for helping to regulate heart rate, blood pressure, and other functions.

Cell cycle. Each cell in the body, including a cancer cell, goes through several stages every time it divides. Various anticancer drugs affect the cell at different stages of this cycle.

Cell-mediated immunity. Immunity provided by *T cells*.

Cervix. The lower portion of the uterus, which protrudes into the vagina. The Pap test is designed to check this area for cancer.

Chemotherapy. The treatment of any disease with chemicals or drugs; a term mostly used in connection with cancer treatment.

Cholesterol. A fatlike substance found in the brain, nerves, liver, blood, and bile. Synthesized in the liver, cholesterol is essential in a number of bodily functions. Excess cholesterol that has been through the process of oxidization contributes to atherosclerosis and heart disease.

Chronobiology. The study of internal body rhythms in order to map hormonal, nerve, and immune-system cyclical functions. Chronobiologists hope to design disease-prevention and treatment strategies based on these cycles that will work more effectively and more safely than general prescriptions.

Circadian rhythm. The biologic clock in humans based on a twenty-four-hour, sunrise/sunset cycle.

Corticoids. A hormone created by the adrenal glands. Generally speaking, corticoids have powerful effects as anti-inflammatories and are essential for the breakdown of carbohydrates and fats in the body.

Delayed sleep-phase syndrome. A sleep disorder related to insomnia in which those afflicted are unable to fall asleep at the desired clock time, instead going to bed much later at night, sleeping later in the morning, and feeling generally lethargic for several hours after awakening.

Depression. A psycho-emotional state marked by feelings of sadness, despair, lack of worth, and hopelessness. The cause of depression can be hereditary or stem from a hormonal imbalance, particularly of the neurotransmitters dopamine, norepinephrine, and *serotonin*. *Melatonin*'s involvement in depression is the subject of intense investigation.

DHEA. A natural steroid hormone secreted by the adrenal glands in youth and early adulthood. Currently investigated as a potential aging trigger, much like melatonin.

DNA (deoxyribonucleic acid). The genetic material of all living things found mainly in the chromosomes in the nucleus of a cell.

Endocrine system. The system of glands and

other structures that secrete *hormones* into the bloodstream, including the thyroid, adrenal, pituitary, pineal, and pancreas.

Estrogen. A group of female hormones responsible for the development of secondary sex traits and aspects of reproduction. Produced in the ovaries, adrenal glands, testicles, and in fat tissue.

Estrogen-receptor (ER) assay: A test that determines whether the breast cancer in a particular patient is stimulated by the hormone *estrogen*.

Estrogen-receptor-positive breast cancer. A type of breast cancer whose growth and development is triggered by the presence of the hormone *estrogen*.

Fight-or-flight response. The body's response to perceived danger or stress, involving the release of hormones and subsequent rise in heart rate, blood pressure, and muscle tension.

Follicle-stimulating hormone (FSH). A hormone secreted by the pituitary gland that prompts the ovaries to ripen an egg each month.

Free radical. A molecule containing an odd number of electrons, making it highly reactive and, as a result, potentially dangerous to healthy cells.

Growth hormone (GH). A hormone secreted by the pituitary gland instrumental in regulating growth. It is released in bursts, especially during sleep, and is controlled by the central nervous system.

High-density lipoprotein (HDL). A lipid-carrying protein that transports the so-called "good" cholesterol away from the artery walls to the liver.

Homeostasis. The relatively constant state of internal temperature and activity—such as heartbeat, blood pressure, and salt balance—within the body regulated by various sensing, feedback, and control systems.

Hormonal anticancer therapy. A form of therapy that takes advantage of the tendency of some cancers to stabilize or shrink if certain hormones are administered or withdrawn.

Hormone. A chemical produced by the endocrine glands or tissue that, when secreted into body fluids, has a specific effect on other organs and processes. Hormones often are referred to as "chemical messengers," and they influence such diverse activities as growth, sexual development, metabolism, and sleep cycles. Hormones also are instrumental in maintaining the proper internal-chemical and fluid balance.

Immunity. The quality of being highly resistant to a disease or *antigen* after initial exposure and response by the immune system.

Immunotherapy. A method of cancer therapy that stimulates the body's own defense mechanisms to attack cancer cells.

Insomnia. A chronic inability to sleep, or to remain asleep, at night. Caused by a variety of factors, including diet and exercise patterns, emotional stress, and hormonal imbalances.

Interferon. A group of proteins released by cells that have been infected with a *virus* and has the ability to inhibit viral growth. Interferon is active against many different viruses.

Interleukin. Any of eight proteins that control aspects of blood-cell production and the immune response; interleukin-2 is known to stimulate *T cells* and is being investigated for the treatment of cancer and Acquired Immune Deficiency Syndrome.

Jet lag. A common sleep disorder resulting from the de-synchronization of the body clock caused by traveling across several time zones.

LDL (low-density lipoprotein). A protein comprised of fats, large amounts of *cholesterol*, and triglycerides. LDLs are considered risk factors for the development of heart disease.

Lymph. Watery fluid in the lymphatic vessels.

Lymph nodes. Oval-shaped organs roughly the size of a pea, located throughout the body, that act as the immune system's first line of defense against infections and cancer. Lymph nodes produce infection-fighting white blood cells as well as filter out bacteria, foreign substances, and cancer cells.

Macrophage. From the Greek "big" and "eater," a white blood cell that destroys foreign substances and cells. It also cooperates with T cells and B cells in the immune response.

Magnetic resonance imaging (MRI). A method of creating three-dimensional images of the body using a magnetic field and radio waves rather than X rays.

Melatonin. A hormone released into the bloodstream by the *pineal gland*. Melatonin production is stimulated by darkness and inhibited by light. It is known to act as a sleep promoter, antioxidant, and immune-system booster.

Metabolism. The sum of all chemical processes that take place in the body essential to convert food to energy and other substances needed to sustain life.

Metastasis. The spread of cancer from one part of the body to another by way of the lymph system or bloodstream. Cells in the new cancer are like those in the original tumor.

Neurotransmitter. A chemical that changes or results in the sending of nerve signals. Neurotransmitters include *serotonin*, *norepinephrine*, and acetylcholine.

Norepinephrine. A so-called stress hormone that, when released, raises blood pressure and rate. Secreted by the adrenal glands.

Oncogenes. Specific stretches of cellular DNA

that, when triggered, contribute to the transformation of normal cells into malignant ones.

Oncologist. A physician who specializes in cancer therapy. There are surgical, radiation, pediatric, gynecological, and medical oncologists. The term *oncologist* alone generally refers to medical oncologists, who are internists with expertise in chemotherapy and the handling of the general medical problems that arise during the disease.

Osteoporosis. A loss of bone density that occurs as a result of calcium and magnesium imbalances in middle to old age. Osteoporosis causes increased porousness and brittleness in the bones.

Pineal gland. The hormone gland located in the brain that secretes *melatonin*. The pineal gland eventually begins to shrink and calcify during the aging process, thereby significantly reducing the amount of circulating melatonin.

Progesterone. A hormone secreted by the adrenals and ovaries. It rises during the second phase of the menstrual cycle.

Prognosis. A statement about the likely outcome of disease in a particular patient based on all available information about that disease, its stage, treatment options, expected results, and other factors.

Prozac. An antidepressant compound that works to block the uptake of the neurotransmitter *se-*

rotonin. Its generic name is fluoxetine hydrochloride.

REM sleep. Rapid-eye movement sleep, the stages of sleep in which dreaming takes place. There generally are four to six REM sleep stages per night, each lasting from a few minutes to half an hour.

Seasonal Affective Disorder (SAD). A mood disorder characterized by mental *depression* related to a certain season of the year, particularly winter. Symptoms include daytime drowsiness and fatigue, diminished concentration, and general lethargy. Some scientists link SAD to overproduction of the hormone *melatonin* due to the long hours of wintertime darkness.

Serotonin. A naturally occurring neurotransmitter derived from the amino acid *tryptophan*.

Stress. Any factor—physical or emotional—that has an effect on the body.

Tamoxifen. A drug that counters the effects of *estrogen* and is used to treat advanced breast cancer in premenopausal women whose tumors are *estrogen-dependent*.

T cells. White blood cells that mature in the thymus and that assist cellular immune reactions.

Testosterone. A naturally occurring hormone responsible for the development of male sex characteristics.

T helper cells. Those *T cells* that assist *B cells* in maturing to produce *antibodies*.

T-suppressor cells. A subclass of *T cells* that suppresses the action of *B cells* to become *antibody* producers and to cause other immune responses.

Thymus gland. A small endocrine gland located in the upper chest that regulates the development of T cells and makes hormones that are important in maintaining a strong, healthy immune system.

Toxin. Any poisonous substance that has the potential to cause disease.

Tryptophan. An essential amino acid used to produce both *serotonin* and *melatonin*. Found in foods such as legumes, grains, and other sources of protein.

Vitamin. Any of a group of substances required by the body for healthy growth, development, and cell repair.

Virus. A tiny particle of *DNA* that is capable of growth only within the nucleus of a cell. Viruses cause any number of diseases, including influenza, the common cold, and more serious conditions, such as AIDS and polio.

References

CHAPTER ONE

Angiers, Natalie. "Modern life suppresses an ancient body rhythm." *The New York Times.* p. C1, March 14, 1995.

Dawson, D. and Encel, N. "Melatonin and sleep in humans." *Journal of Pineal Research.* 1993.

Elias, Marilyn. "The Mysteries of Melatonin." *Harvard Health Letter.* p. 6(3), June 1993.

Haimov, I., Laudon, M., Zisapel, N., Souroujon, M. Nof, D., *et. al.* "Sleep disorders and melatonin rhythms in elderly people." *British Medical Journal.* V. 309, July 16, 1994.

Murray, Frank. Insomnia. *Better Nutrition for Today's Living.* pp. 42-45, June 1994.

Reiter, R.J. "Neuroendocrine effects of light (Review)." *International Journal of Biometeorology.* 35(3): 169-75, Nov. 1991.

Short, R.V. Melatonin. "Melatonin." (Editorial).

British Medical Journal. V. 302: Oct. 16, 1993. p. 952(2).

Thorpy, Michael J., M.D., and Yager, Jan, Ph.D. *The Encyclopedia of Sleep and Sleep Disorders.* New York: Facts on File, 1991.

CHAPTER TWO

Armstrong, S.M., Redman, J.R. "Melatonin: a chronobiotic with anti-aging properties?" *Medical Hypotheses.* 34:300-309, 1991.

". . . But quenched by ubiquitous hormone" (Brain secretion protects oxygen damage to tissues). *Science News*, V. 144, p. 109(1) Aug. 14, 1993.

Davis, W. Marvin. "Health problems of aging." *Drug Topics.* V. 130: p. 98(10), Sept. 5, 1994.

Dori, D., Casale, G. Solerte, S.B., *et.al.* "Chrono-neuroendrocinological aspects of physiological aging and senile dementia." *Chronobiologia.* 21:121-6, Jan.-June 1994.

Grad, B.R., Rozencwaig, R. "The role of melatonin and serotonin in aging: update." *Psychoneuroendicrinology.* 18:283-95, 1993.

Lang, E., Arnold, K., Kupfer, P. "Women live longer: Biological, medical, and sociological causes." *Zeitschrift fur Gerontologie.* 27(1): 10-15, Jan.-Feb. 1994.

Lewis, Alan E. "Actions and uses of melatonin and melatonin with accessory factors (Part 1 and 2)." *Townsend Letter for Doctors.* pp. 1189-1192, 1357-1364, Nov.-Dec. 1994.

Neiman, David C. "It's never too late . . . to change lifestyle habits, that is. *Vibrant Life.* 10:10-12, Nov.-Dec. 1994.

Pierpaoli, W. and Lesnikov, V.A. "The pineal aging clock: Evidence, models, mechanisms, and interventions." *New York Academy of Science*. V. 719, 45-460, 1994.

Pierpaoli, W. and Maestroni, G.J.M. "Melatonin: A principal neuroimmunoregulatory and anti-stress hormone, its anti-aging effects." *Immunology*. 16:355-362, 1987.

Poeggler, B., et. al. "Melatonin, hydroxyl radical-mediated oxidative damage, and aging: A hypothesis." *Journal of Pineal Research*. 14:151-168, 1993.

Vaillant, G.E. "The association of ancestral longevity with successful aging." *Journal of Gerontology*. 46(6): 292-8, Nov. 1991.

Waldhauser, F., Stager H. "Changes in melatonin secretion with age and pubescence." *Journal of Neural Transmission*. 21:183, 1986.

CHAPTER THREE

Cassone, V.M. "Melatonin: Time in a bottle." *Oxford Review of Reproductive Biology*. 12: 319-67, 1990.

Goodwin, Frederick K. "Hickory dickory dock: Who's inherited mousie's clock." *The Journal of the American Medical Association*. V. 267: p. 480(1), Jan. 22, 1992.

Iyengar, B. "Indoleamines and the UV-light-sensitive photoperiodic responses of the melanocyte network: a biological calendar?" *Experientia*. 50(8): 733-6, Aug. 15, 1994.

Levine, Robert L., Pepe, Paul E., Fromm, Robert E., Curko, Peter A., Clark, Peter A. "Prospective evidence of a circadian rhythm for out-of-hospital cardiac arrests." *The Journal of the American Medical Association.* V. 267: p. 2935(3), June 3, 1992.

Levine, M.E., Milliron, A.N., Duffy, L.K. "Diurnal and seasonal rhythms of melatonin, cortisol, and testosterone in interior Alaska." *Arctic Medical Research.* 53(1) 25-34, Jan. 1994.

Lewy, A.J., Sack, R.L. "The dim light: Melatonin onset as a marker for circadian phase position." *Chronobiological Institute.* 8:93-102, 1989.

Maldonano, G., Kraus, J.F. "Variations in suicide occurrence by time of day, day of week, month, and lunar phase." *Suicide Life & Threatening Behavior.* 21:174-87, 1991.

Muller, J.E., Stern, M.D., *et. al.* "Circadian variation in the frequency of onset of acute myocardial infarction." *New England Journal of Medicine.* 313:1315-22, 1985.

Nakagawa, H., Sack, R.L., Lewy, A.J. "Sleep propensity free-runs with the temperature, melatonin, and cortisol rhythms in a totally blind person." *Sleep.* 15(4): 330-6, Aug. 1992.

Rojansky, N., Brzezinski, A., Schenker, J.G. "Seasonality in human reproduction: An update." *Human Reproduction.* 7(6): 735-45, July 1992.

Short, R.V. "Melatonin" (Editorial). *British Medical Journal.* p. 952 (2), Oct. 16, 1993.

Stokkan, K.A., Reiter, R.J. "Melatonin rhythms in Arctic biology." *Journal of Pineal Research.* 16 (1): 33-6, Jan. 1994.

Weissbluth, L., Weissbluth, M. "Infant colic: The effect of serotonin and melatonin circadian rhythms on the intestinal smooth muscle." *Medical Hypotheses.* 39(2): 164-7, Oct. 1992.

Whitney, Hunter. "The biological roller coaster:

Chronobiologists study the body's natural rhythms." *Omni*. V. 16: p. 26(1), Feb. 1994.

CHAPTER FOUR

Dricklin, Mark. "Uncovering another nutritional good guy (glutathione)" (Editorial). *Prevention*. p. 17-20, June 1994.

Gey, K.F., *et al.* "Inverse Correlation between plasma vitamin E and mortality from ischemic heart disease in cross-cultural epidemiology." *American Journal of Clinical Nutrition*. 53 (supp.1): 326-335S, Jan. 1991.

Goldemberg, Robert L. "Free radicals." *Drug & Cosmetics Industry*. 153:40-44, Nov. 1993.

Halliwell, Barry. "Free Radicals, antioxidants, and human disease: curiosity, cause, or consequence?" *The Lancet*. 344: 721-725, Sept. 10, 1994.

Hardeland, R., Reiter, R.J., Poeggler, B. Tan, D.X. "The significance of the metabolism of the neurohormone melatonin: Antioxidant protection and formation of bioactive substances." *Neuroscience & Behavioral Reviews*. 17(3): 347-57, Fall 1993.

Ianas, O., Olinescu, R., Badescu, I. "Melatonin involvement in oxidative processes." *Endocrinologie*. 29(3-2): 147-53, 1991.

LaVecchia, C., *et. al.* "Dietary vitamin A and the risk of cervical cancer." *International Journal of Cancer*. 34(3): 319-322, Sept. 1984.

Muller-Wieland D., Behnke B., Koopman K., Krone W. "Melatonin inhibits LDL receptor activity and cholesterol synthesis in freshly isolated human mononuclear leukocytes."

Biochemical & Biophysical Research Communications. 203(1): 416-21, Aug. 30, 1994.

Neumann, Kimberly. Radical advice. *Women's Sports and Fitness.* p. 25, March 1993.

Pieri, C., Marro, M., *et. al.* "Melatonin, a peroxyl radical scavenger more effective than vitamin E." *Life Sciences.* 55(15): 1271-6, 1994.

Poeggler, B., Reiter, R.J., Tan, D.X., Chen, L.D., Manchester, L.C. "Melatonin, hydroxyl radical-mediated oxidative damage, and aging: A hypothesis." *Journal of Pineal Research.* 14(4): 151-68, May 1993.

Reiter, R.J. "Interactions of the pineal hormone melatonin with oxygen-centered free radicals: a brief review." *Brazilian Journal of Medical and Biological Research.* 26(11): 1141-55, Nov. 1993.

Voelker, Rebecca. "A little exercise goes a long way in cardiovascular health." *American Medical News.* p. 10, July 20, 1992.

CHAPTER FIVE

"Boosting Your Immune System." *The University of California, Berkeley Wellness Letter.* p. 4-6, Oct. 1993.

Caroleo, M.C., Doria, G., Nistico, G. "Melatonin restores immunodepression in aged and cyclophosphamide-treated mice." *Annals of the New York Academy of Sciences.* 719: 343-52, May 31, 1994.

Guerrero, J.M., Reiter, R.J. "A brief survey of pineal gland-immune system interrelationships." *Endocrine Research.* 18(2): 91-113, 1992.

Maestroni, G.J. "The immunoendocrine role of

melatonin" (Review). *Journal of Pineal Research*. 14(1): 1-10, Jan. 1993.

Maestroni, G.J., Conti A. "Immuno-derived opioids as mediators of the immuno-enhancing and anti-stress action of melatonin." *Acta Neurologica*. 13(4): 356-60, Aug. 1991.

Morrey, K.M., McLachlan, J.A., Serkin, C.D. Bakouche, O. "Activation of human monocytes by the pineal hormone melatonin." *Journal of Immunology*. 153(6): 2671-80, Sept. 15, 1994.

Persengiev, S., Marinova C., Patchev, V. "Steroid hormone receptors in the thymus: A site of immunomodulatory action of melatonin." International Journal of Biochemistry. 2(12): 1483-5, 1991.

Pioli C., Caroleo, M.C., Nistico, G. Doria, G. "Melatonin increases antigen presentation and amplifies specific and nonspecific signals for T-cell proliferation." *International Journal of Immunopharmacology*. 15(4): 463-8, May 1993.

Willensky, Diana. "The lymphatic system." *American Health*. p. 82-84, Oct. 1994.

CHAPTER SIX

Ekman, A.C., Leppaluoto, J. Huttunen, P. Aranko, K., Vakkuri, O. "Ethanol inhibits melatonin secretion in healthy volunteers in a dose-dependent randomized double-blind crossover study." *Journal of Clinical Endocrinology & Metabolism*. 77(3): 780-3, Sept. 1993.

Fonzi, S., Solinas, G.P., Costelli, P. *et.al*. "Melatonin and cortisol secretion during ethanol withdrawal in chronic alcoholics." *Chronobiologia*. 21(1-2): 109-12, Jan.-June 1994.

"For men of child-bearing age" (importance of vitamin C). *Tufts University Diet & Nutrition Letter.* p. 1(2), June 1992.

Garland, F.C., *et. al.* "Occupational sunlight exposure and melanoma in the U.S. Navy." *Archives of Environmental Health.* 45: 261-267, 1990.

Goulart, Frances Sheridan. "What's your youth potential?" *Vibrant Life.* p. 19 (1), Jan.-Feb. 1993.

Loscher, W., Wahnschaffe, M., Mevissen, Lerchel, A., Stamm A. "Effects of weak alternating magnetic fields on nocturnal melatonin production and mammary carcinogenesis in rats." (Adapted from *Oncology*, May-June, 1994.) *Cancer Researcher Weekly*, 1: p. 23, June 29, 1994.

Monteleone, P., Maj, M., Fushino, A., Kemali, D. "Physical stress in the middle of the dark phase does not affect light-depressed plasma-melatonin levels in humans." *Neuroendrocrinology.* 55(4): 367-71, April 1992.

Murphy, P.J., Badia, P., Myers, B.L., Boecker, M.R., Wright, K.P. "Nonsteroidal anti-inflammatory drugs affect normal sleep patterns in humans." *Physiology & Behavior.* 55 (6): 1063-6, June 1994.

Reiter, R.J. "Static and extremely low-frequency electromagnetic filed exposure: Reported effects on the circadian production of melatonin." *Journal of Cellular Biology.* 51(4): 394-403, April 1993.

Reiter, R.J., Richardson, B.A. "Some perturbations that disturb the circadian melatonin rhythym." *Chronobiology International.* 9(4): 14-21, Aug. 1992.

Roos, P.A. "Light and electromagnetic waves: The health implications." *The International Journal of Biosocial Research*. 7-10:1-131, 1985-1988.

Sandyk, R. "Magnetic fields in the therapy of parkinsonism" (Review). *International Journal of Neuroscience*. 66(3-4): 209-35, Oct. 1992.

Sandyk, R. Anninos, P.A., Tsagas, N. "Age-related disruption of circadian rhythms: Possible relationship to memory impairment and implications for therapy with magnetic fields" (Review). *International Journal of Neuroscience*. 59(4): 259-62, Aug. 1991.

Schiffman, J.S., Lasch, H.M., Rollag, M.D, *et. al.* "Effect of MR imaging on the normal human pineal body: Measurement of plasma-melatonin levels." *Journal of Magnetic Resonance Imaging*. 4(1) 7-11, Jan.-Feb. 1994.

Schwart, Paul J., Sagan, L. A. "Electromagnetic fields and circadian rhythms." *Journal of the American Medical Association*. p. 868(2), Feb. 17, 1993.

Stevens, R.G. "Biologically based epidemiological studies of electric power and cancer." *Environmental Health Perspectives*. 4:93-100, Dec. 1993.

Tarquini, B., Perfetto, F., Poli R., Tarquini, R. "Daytime circulating melatonin levels in smokers." *Tumori*. 80(3): 229-32, June 30, 1994.

Weber, Karen. "Are you in tune with your body rhythms?" *Current Health*. p. 4(2), April 2, 1993.

Whitaker, J. "Act now to protect your health." *Health and Healing*. Sept. 1993.

Yaga, K., Reiter, R.J., Manchester, *et.al.* "Pineal sensitivity to pulsed static-magnetic fields changes during the photoperiod." *Brain Research Bulletin*, 30(1-2): 153-156, 1993.

CHAPTER SEVEN

Armstrong, S.M., Redman, J.R., "Melatonin: A Chronobiotic with Anti-Aging Properties?" *Medical Hypotheses*. 34:300-309, Aug. 1990.

Iguchi, H., Kato, K. Ibayashi, H. "Age-dependent reduction in serum melatonin concentrations in healthy human subject." *Journal of Clinical and Endocrinological Metabolism*. 55:2, 1982.

Vilijoen, M. Steyn, M.E., et al. "The use of melatonin." *Nephron*. 60:138-143, Jan. 1990.

CHAPTER EIGHT

Bell, David S.H. "The graveyard shift." *Diabetes Forecast*. 47: 46-50, Feb. 1994.

Calverly, P.M.A., Shapiro, C. M. "Medical problems during sleep." *British Medical Journal*. 300: 1403 (3), May, 22, 1993.

Coleman, Daniel. "Too little, too late." *American Health*. p. 43(4), May 1992.

Dahlitz, J., Alvarez, B. Vignau, J., et. al. "Delayed sleep-phase syndrome response to melatonin." *Lancet*. 337: 1121-4, 1991.

"Dieting affects nocturnal body temperature and sleep patterns." *Nutrition Research Newsletter*. 13: 35(1), March 1994.

Gutfeld, Greg. "The new science of rays and rhythms." *Prevention*. 45: 66 (13), Feb. 1993.

"Hormone pills found to fight insomnia." *The New York Times*. p. C8. March 1, 1994.

Koller, M. "Health risks related to shift work." *International Archives of Occupational and Environmental Health.* 53:59, 1983.

Levine, David. "Nature's sleeping pill?" *American Health.* 1:34 (1), July-Aug. 1994.

"Light sleepers." *The Economist.* p. 85 (2), April 11, 1992.

Murphy, P.J., Badia, P., *et. al.* "Nonsteroidal anti-inflammatory drugs affect normal sleep patterns in humans." *Physiology and Behavior.* 55(6): 1063-6, June 1994.

Pavel, S., Goldstein, R., Petruscu, M. "Vasotocin, melatonin, and narcolepsy: Possible involvement of the pineal gland in its patho-physiological mechanism." *Peptides,* 1:281-4, 1980.

Petrie, K., Dawson, A.G., *et. al.* "A double-blind trial of melatonin as a treatment for jet lag in international cabine crew." *Biological Psychiatry.* 33: 526-30, 1993.

Shapiro, G.M., Flanigan, M.J. "Function of sleep." *British Medical Journal.* 300:03 (3), Feb. 8, 1993.

Waldhauser, F., Saletu, B., Trinchard-Lugan, I. "Sleep laboratory investigations on hypnotic properties of melatonin." *Psychopharmachology.* 100:222-6, 1990.

CHAPTER NINE

Checkley, S.A., Murphy, D.G., *et. al.* "Melatonin rhythms in seasonal affective disorder." *British Journal of Psychiatry.* 16: 332-7, Sept. 1993.

Fieve, Ronald, R., M.D. *Prozac: Questions and Answers for Patients, Family, and Physicians.* New York: Avon Books, 1994.

Gutfeld, Greg. "The new science of rays and rhythms." *Prevention.* 45: 66 (3), Feb. 1993.

Mills, M.H., Faunce, T.A. "Melatonin supplementation from early morning auto-urine drinking" (Review). *Medical Hypotheses.* 36 (3): 159-9, Nov. 1991.

Modai, I., Malmgren, R., Wetterberg, L., *et. al.* "Blood levels of melatonin, serotonin, cortisol, and prolactin in relation to the circadian rhythm of platelet serotonin uptake." *Psychiatry Research.* 43(2): 161-6, Aug. 1992.

Rao, M.L., Gross, G., *et. al.* "Circadian rhythm of tryptophan, serotonin, melatonin, and pituitary hormones in schizophrenia." *Biological Psychiatry.* 35: 151-63, Feb. 1, 1994.

Sandyk, R., Awerbuch, G.I. "Multiple sclerosis: The role of the pineal gland in its timing of onset and risk of psychiatric illness." *International Journal of Neuroscience.* 72(1-2): 95-106, Sept. 1993.

Sandyk, R., Tsagas, N., Anninos, P.A. "Melatonin as a proconvulsive hormone in humans." *International Journal of Neuroscience.* 63(1-2): 125-35, March 1992.

Sandyk, R. "The pineal gland and the clinical course of multiple sclerosis." *International Journal of Neuroscience.* 62(1-2): 65-7, Jan. 1992.

Sandyk R., Kay, S.R. "Abnormal EEG and calcification of the pineal gland in schizophrenia." *International Journal of Neuroscience.* 62 (1-2): 107-11, Jan. 1992.

Sandyk, R. "The influence of the pineal gland on migraine and cluster headaches and the effects of treatment with picoTesla magnetic fields." *International Journal of Neuroscience.* 67(1-4): 145-71, Nov.-Dec. 1992.

CHAPTER TEN

Coleman, M.P., Reiter, R.J. "Breast cancer, blindness, and melatonin." *European Journal of Cancer*. 28(2-3): 501-3, 1992.

Furuya, Y., Yamamoto, K., *et. al.* "5-fluorouracil attenuates an oncostatic effect of melatonin on estrogen-sensitive human breast cancer cells." *Cancer Letters*. 81(1): 95-8, June 15, 1994.

Gutfeld, G. "The new science of rays and rhythms." *Prevention*. 45: 66 (3), Feb. 1993.

Hill, S.M., Spriggs, L.L., *et.al.* "The growth inhibitory action of melatonin on human breast-cancer cells is linked to the estrogen-response system." *Cancer Letters*. 64(3): 249-56, July 10, 1992.

Kerenyi, E., Pandula, E., Feuer, G. "Why the incidence of cancer is increasing: The role of light pollution." *Medical Hypotheses*. 33: 75-78, 1990.

Neri, B., Fiorello, C., Moroni, F., *et. al.* "Modulation of human lyphoblastoid interferon activity by melatonin in metastatic renal cell carcinoma: A Phase I study." *Cancer*. 7: 3015(5), June 15, 1994.

Lissoni, P., Barni, S., *et. al.* "A randomized study with the pineal hormone melatonin versus supportive care alone in patients with brain metastases due to solid neoplasms." *Cancer*. 73: 669(3), Feb. 1, 1994.

Lissoni, P., Barni, S., Rovelli, F., *et. al.*, "Neuroimmunotherapy of advanced solid neoplasms with single evening subcutaneous injection of low-dose interleukin-2 and melatonin: Preliminary results." *European Journal of Cancer*. 29A(2): 185-9, 1993.

Lissoni, P., Barni, S., *et. al.* "A study of the mechanisms involved in the immunostimulatory action of the pineal hormone in cancer patients." *Oncology.* 50(6): 399-402, Nov.-Dec. 1993.

Lissoni, P., Barni, S. *et. al.* "Efficacy of the concommitant administration of the pineal hormone melatonin in cancer immunotherapy with low-dose IL-2 in patients with advanced solid tumors who had progressed on IL-2 alone." *Oncology.* 51(4): 3-7, July-Aug. 1994.

Lissoni, P., Barni S., Cattaneo, G., *et. al.* Clinical results with the pineal hormone in advanced cancer resistant to standard anti-tumor therapies." *Oncology.* 48(6): 448-50, 1991.

Sandyk R., Anastasiadis, P.G., Anninos, P.A., Tsagas, N. "Is the pineal gland involved in the pathogenesis of endometrial cancer?" *International Journal of Neuroscience.* 62(1): 89-96, Jan. 1992.

Sankila, R., Joensuu, H., Pukkala, E., Toikkanen, S. "Does the month of diagnosis affect survival of cancer patients?" *British Journal of Cancer.* 67(4): 838-41, April 1993.

CHAPTER ELEVEN

Chiba, A., Akema T., Toyoda, J. "Effects of pinealectomy and melatonin on the timing of proestrus luteinizing hormone surge in the rat." *Neuroendrocrinology.* 59(2): 163-8, Feb. 1994

Coleman, M.P., Reiter, R.J. "Breast cancer, blindness, and melatonin." *European Journal of Cancer.* 28(2-3): 501-3, 1992.

Elias, Marilyn. "The mysteries of melatonin." *Harvard Health Letter*. p. 6(3) June, 1993.

"New breast cancer test." *Cancer Weekly*. March 8, 1993, p. 12.

Reiter, R.J. "The pineal and its hormones in the control of reproduction in mammals." *Endocrine Reviews*. 1:109, 1980.

Porkka-Heiskanen, T. Laskso, M.L., Stenberg, D. "Increase in testosterone sensitivity induced by constant light in relation to melatonin injection in rats." *Journal of Reproduction and Fertility*. 96(1): 331-6, Sept. 1992

Sandyk, R., Anastasiadis, P.G., *et al.* "Is postmenopausal osteoporosis related to pineal gland functions?" *International Journal of Neuroscience*. 62(3-4): 215-25, Feb. 1992.

Silman, R.E. "Melatonin: a contraceptive for the nineties." *European Journal of Obstetrics, Gynecology & Reproductive Biology*. 49(1-2): 3-9, April 1993.

Suzuki, S. Dennerstein, L., Greenwood, K.M., *et al.* "Melatonin and hormonal changes in disturbed sleep during late pregnancy." *Journal of Pineal Research*. 15(4): 191-8, Nov. 1993.

CHAPTER TWELVE

Anonymous. "The Right Time: Chronopharmacology—a new science." *Nursing RSA*. 7(10): 23, 26-27, Oct. 1992

Braverman, Eric R. "DHEA and adrenopause: a new sign of aging and a new treatment." *Total Health*. 10:42(1), Feb. 1994.

Brock, M.A. "Chronobiology and aging." *Journal*

of the American Geriatrics Society 39(1): 74-91, Jan. 1991.

Darrach, Brad. "The war on aging." *Life.* 15:32 (11), Oct. 1992.

Guidici-Fettner, Ann. "DHEA gets respect." *Harvard Health Letter.* 10: 1-3, July 1994.

Halberg, F., Cornelissen, G. Caradente, F. "Chronobiology meets the need for integration in a reductionist climate of biology and medicine." *Chronobiologia.* 18(2-3): 93-103, Apr.-Sept. 1991.

Whitney, Hunter. "The biological roller coaster: chronobiologists study the body's natural rhythms." *Omni.* 18:28. Feb. 1994.

Index

M

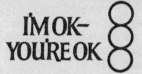

COMPREHENSIVE,
AUTHORITATIVE
REFERENCE WORKS
FROM AVON TRADE BOOKS

THE OXFORD AMERICAN DICTIONARY
Edited by Stuart Berg Flexner, Eugene Ehrlich and
Gordon Carruth
51052-9/ $12.50 US/ $15.00 Can

THE CONCISE COLUMBIA DICTIONARY
OF QUOTATIONS
Robert Andrews
70932-5/ $9.95 US/ $11.95 Can

THE CONCISE COLUMBIA ENCYCLOPEDIA
Edited by Judith S. Levey and Agnes Greenhall
63396-5/ $14.95 US

THE NEW COMPREHENSIVE AMERICAN
RHYMING DICTIONARY
Sue Young
71392-6/ $12.00 US/ $15.00 Can

KIND WORDS: A THESAURUS
OF EUPHEMISMS
Judith S. Neaman and Carole G. Silver
71247-4/ $10.95 US/ $12.95 Can

THE WORLD ALMANAC GUIDE
TO GOOD WORD USAGE
Edited by Martin Manser with Jeffrey McQuain
71449-3/ $8.95 US